Tinnitus

A multidisciplinary approach

GERHARD ANDERSSON PhD
Linköping University

DAVID M BAGULEY MSc, MBA
Addenbrookes Hospital NHS Trust, Cambridge

LAURENCE MCKENNA PhD, M Clin Psychol
Royal National Throat, Nose and Ear Hospital, London

DON MCFERRAN MA, FRCS
Essex County Hospital, Colchester

W
WHURR PUBLISHERS
LONDON AND PHILADELPHIA

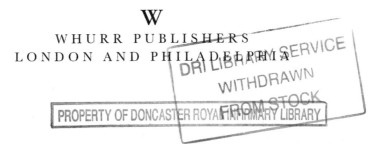

© 2005 Whurr Publishers Ltd
First published 2005 by Whurr Publishers
19b Compton Terrace, London N1 2UN, England and
325 Chestnut Street, Philadelphia PA 19106, USA

British Library Cataloguing in Publication data

A catalogue record for this book is available from the British
Library.

ISBN 1 86156 403 1

Printed and bound in the UK by Athenaeum Press Limited,
Gateshead, Tyne & Wear.

Contents

Acknowledgements   viii
Foreword   ix
  Professor Richard Tyler, University of Iowa
Preface   xi

Chapter 1   1

Introduction

Chapter 2   14

Prevalence and natural history

Chapter 3   25

Mechanisms

Chapter 4   35

Medical models of tinnitus

Chapter 5   55

Psychological and neurophysiological models of tinnitus

Chapter 6   63

How tinnitus is perceived and measured

Chapter 7   71

Objective correlates of tinnitus

Chapter 8   **82**

Self-report and interview measures of tinnitus severity and impact

Chapter 9   **93**

Consequences and moderating factors

Chapter 10   **112**

Hyperacusis

Chapter 11   **123**

Traditional treatments

Chapter 12   **135**

Tinnitus retraining therapy

Chapter 13   **145**

A cognitive behavioural treatment programme

Chapter 14   **159**

Complementary medicine approaches to tinnitus

Chapter 15   **166**

A multidisciplinary synthesis

References   **171**
Index   **205**

Dedication

This book is dedicated with love to Ebba and Edvin Andersson, Bridget and Sheila Baguley, Tanya McFerran and Anne O'Sullivan

Acknowledgements

Grateful thanks are due to Lucy Handscomb and Professor Dafydd Stephens, for being diligent critical readers, and to Dr Dave Furness, Keele University, for generosity with electromicrographs.

Foreword

Many clinicians do not know how to help tinnitus patients. Their coursework on tinnitus and their clinical experience with tinnitus patients may be limited. They may feel threatened by the patient, or they may not be sure they can actually help the patient. Clinicians may have been trained on one particular approach, but may not feel confidence about it. Some tinnitus patients present with severe anxiety and inappropriate coping strategies; some are desperate and susceptible to unfounded, often expensive, treatments. Few clinicians have a strong background in both hearing and counselling. Where do we start?

Treating tinnitus can involve many disciplines and many professionals. Audiologists, otologists, clinical psychologists and hearing therapists, as well as primary care physicians and nurses, are often involved. Tinnitus research has also risen to the foreground in a wide range of scientific disciplines.

The rationale for this book, *Tinnitus: A multidisciplinary approach*, is to provide a broad and detailed account of recent developments in tinnitus research and clinical management. It represents a collaborative effort to summarize the current literature and to offer new perspectives. Gerhard Andersson (Professor of Clinical Psychology), David Baguley (Consultant Audiological Scientist), Laurence McKenna (Consultant Clinical Psychologist) and Don McFerran (Consultant Otolaryngologist) are to be congratulated for this significant contribution to the field of tinnitus. The authors have much experience in providing both clinical service and performing research on tinnitus. The book is unique in the broad range of topics covered, and is supported by an extensive list of references. The style is straightforward and easy to read. It truly presents a multidisciplinary approach, including audiological, neuroscience, medical and psychological perspectives. Further, the authors include practical advice on how to assess and treat tinnitus patients.

Knowledge represents the essential foundation to be able to provide effective treatments. You hold in your hands a valuable tool that reviews much of the important information about tinnitus. Enjoy reading it, knowing that you will become a better clinician.

Richard S Tyler
University of Iowa

Preface

While there has been much scientific and clinical enquiry about tinnitus, it continues to be a fascinating and enigmatic phenomenon. This book aims to present current understandings on tinnitus from a multidisciplinary perspective. In fact, we believe that it is only through the convergence of knowledge from neuroscience, audiology, otology, pharmacology and psychology that progress will be made in developing and delivering truly effective treatments.

Thus, in a very real sense, this book represents the book the authors wish had been available when they began their involvement with tinnitus patients. Historical and current perspectives on tinnitus are presented, with careful and critical reflection. Treatment paradigms are reviewed in the light of conceptual underpinnings and of available clinical evidence.

The writing of the book has been a rewarding and challenging process, and it has mirrored our tinnitus careers. Just as we have interwoven our experience and knowledge in the manuscript, so have the four of us found ourselves interwoven in training, in clinical work, in research and in friendship. It is our hope that our collaboration of authorships will inform and inspire present and future tinnitus clinicians and researchers, and that their achievements may far surpass what is presently available.

There are so many colleagues and mentors who have supported, encouraged and sometimes cajoled us in our tinnitus work that to list them would not be practical. They are all thanked, as are our families, who have borne with our tinnitus obsessions. Finally, we thank our patients, who have tolerated our learning curves, experiments, enquiries and our attempts to treat them.

Gerhard Andersson
David Baguley
Laurence McKenna
Don McFerran

Chapter 1
Introduction

Tinnitus and hyperacusis continue to intrigue patients, scientists and clinicians alike. That so many people can have some experience of these symptoms and not be distressed, whilst others are troubled to the point that they are no longer able to perform their normal daily activities remains paradoxical. Furthermore, the fact that when tinnitus is matched in intensity in this troubled group of people, it has consistently been reported to be of lower subjective intensity than a whisper. Despite this low intensity the intrusiveness of the symptom in patients with severe tinnitus is remarkable. Given these paradoxes, it is unsurprising that no single approach to tinnitus and hyperacusis has been shown to be overwhelmingly stronger than any other in terms of understanding tinnitus and hyperacusis and of managing these symptoms.

The aim of this book is to present a multidisciplinary approach to tinnitus and hyperacusis, incorporating insights from audiology, otology, psychology, psychiatry and auditory neuroscience. It is hoped that this will inspire a collaborative approach to tinnitus and hyperacusis management that will benefit patients and clinicians alike. There is already good evidence that such collaborative and multidisciplinary initiatives in the field of chronic pain have increased the efficacy of treatments.

Definitions

The word *tinnitus* derives from the Latin verb 'tinnire' meaning 'to ring', and in common English usage is defined as 'a ringing in the ears' (*Concise Oxford English Dictionary*; Allen, 1990). The first recorded in use of the word occurred in 1693, in Blanchard's *Physician's Dictionary*, second edition, as follows:

> Tinnitus Aurium, a certain buzzing or tingling in the Ears proceding from obstruction, or something that irritates the Ear, whereby the Air that is shut up is continually moved the beating of the Arteries, and the Drume of the Ear is lightly verberated, whences arises a Buzzing and a Noife. (Stephens, 2000: 201)

1

Some other languages have a variety of words to describe this phenomenon (Stephens, 2000), notably French where five words are in regular use, each describing a particular timbre or quality of sound. In Swedish the word for tinnitus used to be öronsus, which in direct translation stands for 'ear breeze'. Few patients would agree that their tinnitus sounds like a breeze. In an attempt at a scientific definition McFadden (1982) considered that 'Tinnitus is the conscious expression of a sound that originates in an involuntary manner in the head of its owner, or may appear to him to do so.' and this definition has been widely adopted (e.g. Coles, 1987; Davis and El Rafaie, 2000; Stephens, 2000).

Definitions of hyperacusis have tended to illustrate the perspective of the author. For instance, Vernon (1987b) proposed an open definition as 'unusual tolerance to ordinary environmental sounds', but far more perjorative is that of Klein et al. (1990), 'consistently exaggerated or inappropriate responses or complaints to sounds that are neither intrinsically threatening or uncomfortably loud to a typical person'.

Attempts have been made more recently to differentiate between those individuals who have a general hypersensitivity to sound that others can tolerate (hyperacusis), and those who find specific sounds uncomfortable, perhaps because of emotional associations with that sound. In an initial differentiation between these two, the second experience was entitled 'phonophobia', a term that is commonly used in neurology (Woodhouse and Drummond, 1993), in particular in association with migraine attacks. However, the inference that this phenomenon was essentially phobic in nature can be unhelpful to some patients. Definitions of hyperacusis are further explored in Chapter 10.

Historical aspects

The experience of the perception of sound generated internally has been mentioned in many historical medical texts. These original sources have been reviewed by Stephens (1987, 2000) and Feldmann (1997), and whilst these authors have many detailed issues upon which they are at variance with one another, they are in broad agreement on the interest expressed in tinnitus by medical authors from historical times. A series of ancient Babylonian medical texts, inscribed upon clay tablets, was housed in the library of King Assurbanipal (668–626 BC) in Ninevah. These were translated by Thompson (1931) and were found to include 22 references to tinnitus, described variously as the ears 'singing', 'speaking' or 'whispering'. Treatments are described, including whispered incantations, the instillation of various substances into the external auditory meatus and the application of charms (such as the tooth of a female ibex): specific treatments were advised for each experience of tinnitus as described above (Feldmann, 1997). The involvement of ghosts and spirits in the generation of tinnitus was described, and in particular the incantation method of treatment was largely concerned with driving away such affliction, this being described as the basis of much human disease (Stephens, 1987). Tinnitus has six mentions in the *Corpus Hippocratum*, a second-century AD compilation of the works of Hippocrates of Kos (460–377 BC): each mention relates to a description of ear disease rather than of tinnitus as an experience in its own right. Other authors writing in Graeco-Roman times mentioning tinnitus include Celsus (25 BC– 50 AD), who described treatments with diet and abstinence from wine, and Pliny the Elder (23–79 AD), who advocated the use of wild cumin and almond oil in cases of tinnitus (Stephens, 2000). The use of sedative medication to treat people suffering with tinnitus, still in common use in the USA and Western Europe, was first described by Galen (129–199 AD), who considered the benefits of opium and mandrake.

There are mentions of tinnitus in texts within the Islamic medical tradition from the period following the decline of medicine in Rome (Stephens 1987, 2000; Feldmann 1997). These include the first mention of the coincident complaint of tinnitus and hyperacusis by Paul of Aegina (625–690 AD) (Stephens, 2000 after Adams, 1844).

Advances in the understanding and treatment of tinnitus were not to be seen until the seventeenth century, with the publication of the first text entirely dedicated to the ear and hearing. The *Traité de l'Organe de l'Ouie* by DuVerney (1683) was translated from the original French into Latin, German, Dutch and English and is recognized as a milestone in otology (Weir, 1990). The insights into tinnitus represented a move away from the concept that tinnitus may arise from trapped air in the ear, this having persisted since Roman times, towards a model of tinnitus arising from diseases of the ear and disorders of the brain. The implication of the influence of the brain over the ear is prophetic of later concepts of the function of the efferent auditory system in humans. The treatments for tinnitus that are advocated by DuVerney are limited to treatment of the underlying disorder.

A further advance in understanding occurred in 1821 with the publication of *Traité des Malades de l'Oreille et de l'Audition* by Itard. This comprehensive text was based upon 20 years of experience in working with the deaf, and contained numerous case studies, including that of Jean-Jacques Rousseau (1712–1778) the eminent philosopher who became afflicted by tinnitus in later life (Feldmann, 1997). Itard made the distinction between tinnitus experiences arising from sound, thus 'objective tinnitus' such as that caused by somatosounds, and that arising without any acoustic basis, 'false tinnitus'. This distinction is still in use today. In addition to such medical insights Itard described the effect of tinnitus upon an individual: 'an extremely irksome discomfort which leads to a profound sadness in affected individuals.' (translation by Stephens, 2000: 443). The treatment of tinnitus was, as with previous authors, based upon treatment of the underlying otological condition, although when such treatment failed Itard advocated attention to the behavioural manifestation of tinnitus and in particular to sleep disturbance, when the use of external environmental sound (such as a watermill or an open fire burning damp wood) to mask the tinnitus was suggested.

In the late nineteenth century the medical speciality of otology underwent a renewal of interest and effort, and several individuals have been identified as leaders in this field. Joseph Toynbee (1815–1866) and William Wilde (1815–1876) (the father of Oscar Wilde) were pre-eminent in this regard and wrote extensively on ear disease, including consideration of tinnitus arising from such conditions. Toynbee experienced distressing tinnitus himself, and died during an experiment in which he attempted to determine 'the effect of inhalation of chloroform upon tinnitus, when pressed into the tympanum.' (Feldmann, 1997: 18). MacNaughton Jones (1891) has been credited (Stephens, 2000) with producing the first book in English on tinnitus alone, this containing a classification of tinnitus based upon the site of origin and a review of contemporary treatments.

The ability to use electronic instruments to measure hearing accurately by audiometry, and the consequent ability to determine hearing status in patients with a complaint of tinnitus, was developed in the early twentieth century and became widespread in Western Europe and the USA from the 1940s (Weir, 1990). At this time, Fowler (1941) considered the characteristics of tinnitus and is credited with the first comprehensive attempts to determine the matching and masking characteristics of tinnitus (Stephens, 2000). Among the insights gleaned by Fowler were: that subjectively loud tinnitus is often matched to a low-level stimulus; that tinnitus may be masked by a broad-band noise; and that it is not possible to generate beats between tinnitus and externally generated tones (Fowler, 1941). In subsequent writings Fowler collaborated with his son, also an otologist, and formulated a protocol for the examination of tinnitus patients considering the qualities of the sound, the distress associated, as well as the otological health of the patient (Fowler and Fowler, 1955).

This short review of the historical understanding of tinnitus has three underpinning elements. The first is that any consideration of tinnitus and formulation of possible treatment should consider the otological status of the patient and thus involve the treatment of ear disease where indicated. The second is that this otological focus does not relieve the clinician of the responsibility to consider the distress caused by the tinnitus experience, and where significant behavioural manifestation of this is present, to treat that distress. The third is that the understanding and treatment of tinnitus is a changing and developing science.

Anatomy and physiology

The aspects of the human auditory system (Figure 1.1) relevant to an understanding of tinnitus and hyperacusis are now described.

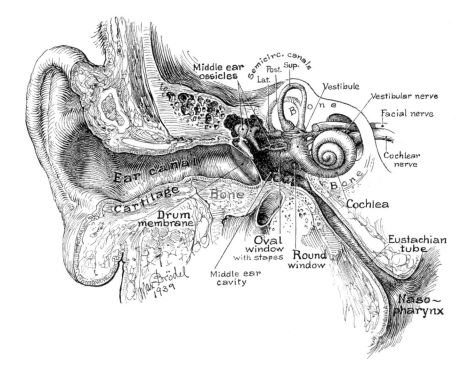

Figure 1.1. The human ear. (From Brodel, 1946, with permission.)

Outer ear

The outer ear consists of the pinna and the external auditory meatus, these structures being lateral to the tympanic membrane. The pinna has a cartilaginous skeleton with some vestigial muscular attachments. The external auditory meatus is between 2 cm and 3 cm long, is 5–9 mm in diameter in adult humans and is oval-shaped. The lateral portion (comprising one-third of the length) is cartilaginous and lined with squamous epithelium rich in cerumen-producing glands and hair. The medial portion (comprising two-thirds of the length) is bony and lined by stratified squamous epithelium. This epithelium is continuous with the tympanic membrane. The external auditory meatus is curved in a slight antero-inferior direction, meeting the tympanic membrane obliquely so that the posterior wall is is shorter and shallower than the anterior wall. The external auditory meatus has a resonant frequency approximating 3000 Hz in the adult human.

Tympanic membrane

The tympanic membrane has three layers comprising: an outer layer continuous with the epithelium of the external auditory meatus; a fibrous middle layer of crossed collagen fibres; and an inner layer of mucous membrane. The rim, or annulus, of the tympanic membrane is approximately circular in shape. The tympanic membrane itself is shaped like a shallow cone (Figure 1.2), drawn in medially to a connection with the malleus. The small central upper portion of the tympanic membrane, above the lateral process of the malleus is called the 'pars flaccida', and unlike the remaining larger 'pars tensa', does not possess a middle fibrous layer.

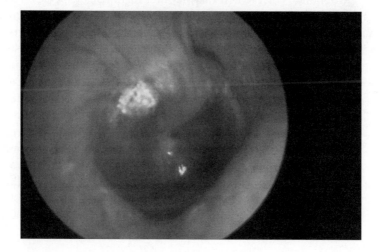

Figure 1.2 The right tympanic membrane.

Middle ear

The middle ear is an impedance-matching transformer. Its function is to change the characteristics of sound vibrations that have passed through air into vibrations that are suitable for passing through the aqueous medium of the inner ear. In structure it is an air-filled space, bounded by the tympanic membrane laterally and medially by the bone covering the inner ear. In addition, this tympanum is connected via a short tunnel (aditus ad antrum) in the area above the tympanic membrane known as the attic to the mastoid antrum, a honeycomb of air cells within the mastoid bone. The tympanum is bridged by the ossicular chain, comprising the malleus, incus and stapes, connected to the tympanic membrane by the malleus and to the labyrinth at the footplate of the stapes. The ossicular chain is suspended within the tympanum by folds of mucous membrane, and controlled in movement by the tensor-tympani muscle, which contracts in conjunction with palatal movement, and by the stapedius, which is innervated by the facial nerve and contracts in response to loud sound (stapedial reflex). The middle ear is ventilated by the Eustachian tube, running in from the anterior portion of the middle ear to the nasopharynx. The Eustachian tube opens with swallowing and yawning, and allows nasally inhaled air to replenish air in the tympanum, which is continuously absorbed by the mucous membrane lining.

Cochlea

The human cochlea consists of a coiled tube within the temporal bone, deriving its name from the Latin *cochlea* (snail). In humans there are 2.75 turns (33 mm in total length), dimensions which vary in other mammalian species. The bony shell of the human cochlea coils around the modiolus, a central bony canal containing the cochlear ganglion. The cochlear labyrinth contains three channels: the scala vestibuli (filled with perilymph and to which the stapes is connected at the stapes footplate); the scala media (filled with endolymph and thus sometimes entitled the endolymphatic space); and the scala tympani (again filled with perilymph). The scalae vestibuli and tympani communicate at the apex of the cochlea via an opening called the heliocotrema.

The scala media is separated from the scala vestibuli by Reissner's membrane, and from the scala tympani by the basilar membrane, and has a triangular shape in cross-section. Set upon the basilar membrane is the Organ of Corti, a complex structure whose micromechanical properties allow the transduction of sound. This is accomplished by approximately 16 000 hair cells within a human cochlea, these being arranged tonotopically and being innervated by a total of 30 000 afferent nerve fibres (Figure 1.3).

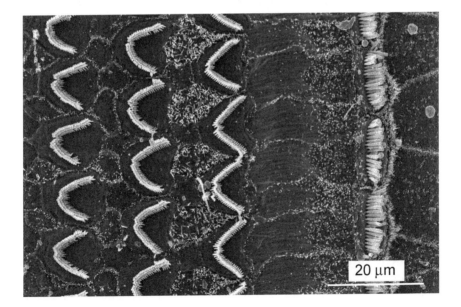

20 μm

Figure 1.3 Scanning electron micrograph of reticular lamina showing three rows of outer hair cells with W-shaped hair bundles and the single row of inner hair cells with more linear bundles. The hair cells are separated by supporting cells. (Micrograph supplied by DN Furness, Keele Unversity and CM Hackney, University of Wisconsin–Madison.)

Of the two varieties of hair cell in the human cochlea the inner hair cells form a single row close to the modiolus and number approximately 3500 in a healthy cochlea. Inner hair cells are flask-shaped with a central nucleus. The innervation of the inner hair cell is predominantly afferent.

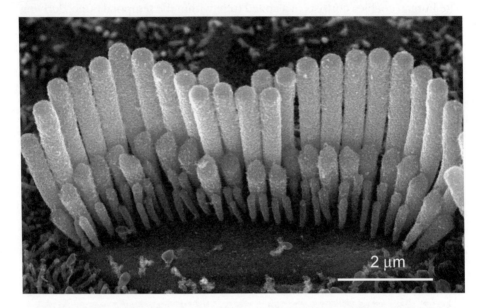

Figure 1.4 Scanning electron micrograph of a single hair bundle from an inner hair cell. (Micrograph supplied by DN Furness, Keele University and CM Hackney, University of Wisconsin–Madison.)

Further from the modiolus the 12 000 outer hair cells are arranged in three rows (Figure 1.5), the space between the inner hair cells and outer hair cells being bounded by pillar cells. Outer hair cells are longer than inner hair cells in humans (30–70 μm in length) and are cylindrical in shape, with a basally located nucleus. A distinctive feature is the large number of mitochondria sited around the sides of outer hair cells, and associated with sub-surface cisternae. Isolated outer hair cells have been demonstrated to have motile properties when subjected to electrical or mechanical stimulation.

The innervation of the outer hair cells is predominantly efferent. The tips of the outer hair cell stereocilia are embedded in the gelatinous tectorial membrane, whereas evidence suggests that those of the inner hair cells are not. The vibration of sound on the basilar membrane causes a travelling wave; the deflection at the point of that travelling wave causing sufficient motion in the inner hair cells to cause depolarization of the hair cell and hence firing of the ganglion.

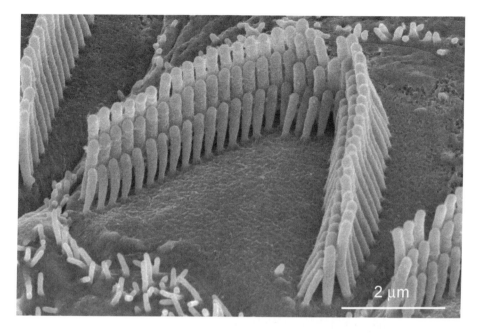

Figure 1.5 Scanning electron micrograph of a single hair bundle from an outer hair cell. Note that the stereocilia are present in three rows, the rows ranked in increasing height across the bundle. (Micrograph supplied by DN Furness, Keele University.)

Spiral ganglion

The spiral ganglion is contained within the modiolus, and contains both Type I ganglion cells, with dendrites entitled 'radial fibres' that synapse with inner hair cells, and the Type II ganglion cells with outer spiral fibre dendrites that synapse with outer hair cells. The tonotopicity of the basilar membrane is evident within the spiral ganglion, in that the fibres associated with hair cells at the apex of the cochlea are found in the centre of the spiral ganglion, whilst those that are associated with hair cells in the basal turn of the cochlea are found at the outside.

Internal auditory canal and cerebellopontine angle

The internal auditory canal is a bony channel for the cochlear and vestibular (VIII) nerves and facial (VII) nerves to progress to the intracranial cavity. In addition, the internal auditory canal contains the nervus intermedius and the labyrinthine artery and vein. Three regions of the internal auditory canal are identified: the fundus (abutting upon the medial aspect of the labyrinth, the lateral boundary of the fundus meeting the dura); the canal proper (the dimensions of which vary with the dimensions of the temporal bone and hence show considerable variation -mean length 8 mm, mean diameter

3.68 mm; Gulya and Schuknecht (1995)); and the porus (located on the posterior surface of the temporal bone).

At the fundus of the internal auditory canal the superior vestibular and facial nerves occupy the superior portion of the canal, with the cochlear and inferior vestibular nerves located inferiorly. The VIIth/VIIIth nerve complex undergoes a 90° rotation as it continues through the internal auditory canal, and at the porus the divisions of the vestibular nerve have merged (this fusion occuring just proximal to the transverse crest) and the cochlear nerve has merged with the vestibular nerve, though the cochlear nerve fibres remain placed inferiorly. The trunks of the cochlear and vestibular nerves remain separated by a septum at the porus, although surgical specimens have shown variability in the completeness of this septum (Gulya and Schuknecht, 1995). The anastomosis of Oort (Oort, 1918) consists of a bundle of fibres running from the saccular branch of the inferior vestibular nerve to the cochlear nerve and contains efferent fibres from the medial olivo-cochlear system (Rasmussen, 1946). This vestibulo-cochlear anastomosis has been measured at 2–3 mm long and 0.1–0.3 mm wide at the base in adult humans (Arnesen, 1984), and consists of both myelinated and unmyelinated axons, with unmyelinated axons in the majority (ratio 3.0:1.0).

The VIIth/VIIIth nerve complex leaves the porus of the internal auditory canal and crosses a region bounded laterally by the medial portion of the posterior surface of the temporal bone, posteriorly by the cerebellar hemisphere and the flocculus, and medially by the pons, entitled the cerebellopontine angle, containing cerebospinal fluid. In an adult human the distance from the porus to the medullary–pontine junction where the vestibulo-cochlear nerve enters the brainstem is 23–24 mm.

Central auditory pathways

The human central auditory pathways form a complex system, with processing at feature extraction evident from a low level, but also with the maintenance of the tonotopicity set up in the cochlea to a cortical level.

Cochlear nucleus

The cochlear nucleus complex spans the ponto–medullary junction, and is divisable into two portions: the dorsal cochlear nucleus and the ventral cochlear nucleus. The ventral cochlear nucleus is further subdivided into the anterior ventral cochlear nucleus and the posterior ventral cochlear nucleus. Each cochlear nerve fibre divides into two main branches at entry to the brainstem, with an ascending branch to the anterior ventral cochlear nucleus, and a descending branch to the posterior ventral cochlear nucleus and thence to the dorsal cochlear nucleus. In each division of the cochlear nucleus complex the tonotopicity set up within the cochlea is maintained, and such apparent redundancy is indicative of processing and feature extraction at this stage. In the anterior ventral cochlear nucleus the ascending branches of Type I spiral ganglion neurones synapse with the end-bulbs of Held, large excitatory terminals with a purely relay function, ensuring the maintenance of precise tonotopicity within the arrangement of spherical busy cells in the anterior ventral cochlear nucleus. The axons of the spherical busy cells are large and myelinated, and leave the anterior ventral cochlear nucleus as the ventral acoustic stria, further entitled the 'trapezoid body' as it approaches the superior olivary complex.

Within the posterior ventral cochlear nucleus and the dorsal cochlear nucleus lie multipolar cells that receive inputs from several cochlear nerve fibres, thus allowing frequency and intensity coding and comparison. Whilst most of the axons from these cells project to the contralateral inferior colliculus, a number send branches to the peri-olivary region associated with the olivo-cochlear efferent system. Also within the posterior ventral cochlear nucleus are located octopus cells, which respond rapidly and that have been associated with startle responses to auditory stimuli.

Superior olivary complex and medial olivo-cochlear bundle

Axons from spherical bushy cells in both ventral cochlear nuclei synapse with neurones in the superior olivary complex. Processing of these binaural inputs with regard to time differences has been associated with the medial superior olive, and with regard to intensity differences with the lateral superior olive (the smaller of the two divisions), both these functions being involved in sound localization for low- and high-frequency sound, respectively.

The peri-olivary nuclei are small and diffuse, surrounding the medial and lateral superior olive. The medial peri-olivary nuclei are collectively described as the medial olivo-cochlear bundle, and consist of large multipolar neurones. The large majority of axons cross the mid-line, and exit the brainstem as an element of the vestibular nerve, specifically within the inferior vestibular division. These efferent fibres leave the inferior vestibular nerve and join the cochlear nerve at the anastomosis of Oort (Oort, 1918) just beyond the saccular ganglion. At this point the efferent pathway consists of about 1300 fibres, 75% of which are unmyelinated (Arnesen, 1984; Schuknecht, 1993) and thence enter the cochlea via the modiolus through Rosenthal's canal to synapse with the outer hair cells. Axons from the ipsilateral olivo-cochlear bundle follow an ipsilateral inferior vestibular nerve route to the inner hair cells within the ipsilateral cochlea.

Inferior colliculus

The inferior colliculi are located on the dorsal surface of the mid-brain and receive branches from the contralateral cochlear nuclei running ventrally through the brainstem via the lateral lemnisci. The role of the inferior colliculi is as vital to audition as is the role of the superior colliculi in vision, and co-ordination of vision and audition is undertaken by connections between these two areas.

The central nucleus of the inferior colliculi is the largest brainstem auditory nucleus, and the tonotopicity seen in lower auditory brainstem structures is maintained. Within the central nuclei of the inferior colliculi, frequency and intensity maps interrelate, as does information about the temporal characteristics of sound. As described above, these maps of auditory information are integrated with visual space map information in the superior colliculi.

Medial geniculate body

Fibres from the inferior colliculi project to each of the three subdivisions (ventral, dorsal and medial) of the auditory nuclei on the surface of the thalamus, the medial geniculate body, though it is the ventral division of the medial geniculate body that receives the majority of fibres. The ventral medial geniculate body is organized tonotopically and projects to the primary auditory cortices, these projections being reciprocated. In contrast, the dorsal and lateral medial geniculate bodies project to the associative auditory cortices, and the medial division in particular is multimodal, containing visual, somatosensory and vestibular information, and a role as a multisensory arousal system has been proposed. The dorsal medial geniculate body has been thought to have a more auditory-specific arousal function.

Auditory and associative cortices

In humans the primary auditory cortices are situated within the lateral fissure of the temporal lobe (Brodmann's areas 41 and 42) and are binaurally innervated, and a significant role in the perception of sound localization is implied. Whilst Brodmann's area 41 has the characteristic structure of primary cortex, Brodmann's area 42, whilst also innervated by the ventral medial geniculate body, has a structure indicative of associative cortex. Information processed by Brodmann's areas 41 and 42 is passed to Brodmann's area 22, the most important of the association auditory cortical areas for speech processing.

Interactions with other systems

Throughout the auditory system there are interactions with other systems, these connections integrating auditory information with that of the other senses, and facilitating the response to such stimuli. The interactions between such systems are complex, and lie outside the scope of this review. Those interactions that are relevant to an understanding of tinnitus, however, are the connections between the auditory system and mechanisms of arousal and behavioural reaction to sound, and between audition and emotional reaction to sound.

The reticular formation is located within the central core of the brainstem, and is so called because of the net-like appearance of the fibre structure when seen in cross-section. This brainstem core is continuous with the intermediate gray matter of the spinal cord caudally and with the lateral hypothalamic and subthalamic regions rostrally. Many functions of the reticular formation have been identified, and this, in conjunction with the diffuse structure of the formation, has led some to question the validity of the term 'reticular formation', preferring to name separate subsystems (see Heimer, 1995 and Saper, 2000 for review). Of interest when considering tinnitus are the functions of the medial reticular formation in mediating the sympathetic autonomic response to auditory stimulation, thus facilitating the behavioural response to alarming or unexpected stimuli (a function also involving the octopus cells of the posterior ventral cochlear nucleus), and of sleep regulation. In the latter case the rostral portion of the reticular formation (above the pons) has been implicated in wakefulness, this activity being normally inhibited by areas of the reticular formation below the pons (Rechtshaffen and Siegel, 2000). Consideration of the restlessness, agitation and sleep disturbance associated with tinnitus has implicated reticular formation responses to tinnitus (Jastreboff, 1990).

Human emotional responses have been considered to involve a system of brain structures entitled the 'limbic system', first described by Papez (1937) and elaborated by MacLean (1955), and including the amygdala, hippocampus and hypothalamus. This initial model has been very significantly elaborated and modified (see LeDoux, 1998 for review), and greater emphasis is placed upon the role of the amygdalae, in particular in experiences of fear and anxiety, whilst the hippocampus is now considered as involved in encoding short-term memory (Iversen et al., 2000). The use of auditory stimuli in experiments concerning animal models of fear conditioning has led to models of interaction between the auditory system and the limbic system, and two main pathways for interaction have been identified. The first is that between associative auditory cortex and the amygdala, and the second between the thalamic auditory nuclei - those being the medial geniculate body and the extralemniscal auditory pathways (LeDoux, 1998). These second interactions have been implicated in the experiences of tinnitus patients of anxiety, apprehension and fear about their tinnitus (Møller et al., 1992; Eggermont, 2000).

Summary

From the above it is evident that concern with tinnitus is not new, and in fact is demonstrated throughout written human history. Additionally, a review of the complex anatomy of the human auditory system and its intimate relationship with systems of reaction, arousal and emotion, indicate that a holistic view of tinnitus must consider the involvement of such systems.

Chapter 2
Prevalence and natural history

The prevalence of tinnitus has been investigated in several studies over the years, but figures vary given differences in the definition and duration of tinnitus. However, an overall approximation suggests that across studies somewhere between 10% and 15% of the population have tinnitus. Another common observation is that only small proportions of all people with tinnitus are troubled by it. This figure ranges between one in ten and one in five. Although gender differences have been observed (for example, women have been reported to have more complex tinnitus sounds than men (Meikle and Greist, 1989; Dineen et al., 1997a)), there are no clear indications why tinnitus should be experienced differently by men and women. Neither are there any consistent differences in prevalence, apart from a small trend for females to be more likely to be affected (Davis and El Rafaie, 2000). The onset of tinnitus is often abrupt, but it is not uncommon that tinnitus onset is insidious. A common finding in the epidemiological literature on tinnitus is that it is more common in unskilled versus professional social classes, and this is not explained purely by differences in noise exposure (Davis and El Rafaie, 2000).

Transient tinnitus is a very common experience (Schulman, 1997), and perhaps so common that it is rarely noticed. It is therefore understandable that this form of tinnitus is excluded from most epidemiological studies. The majority of studies also exclude tinnitus following noise exposure. The most extensive studies on the prevalence of tinnitus have been conducted by Adrian Davis and co-workers at the Institute of Hearing Research in Nottingham, UK (Davis and El Rafaie, 2000). This group developed the term 'prolonged spontaneous tinnitus', which was defined as tinnitus that arose spontaneously rather than in response to noise and lasted longer than five minutes at a time. It is not clear why the five-minute criterion was chosen, but it makes clinical sense as brief transient tinnitus by nature seldom lasts longer than a few seconds.

The literature on the prevalence of tinnitus is not extensive, but is not easy to access, as many studies have not been published in MEDLINE-indexed journals. A MEDLINE search on the key words *tinnitus* and *prevalence* results in many references but most of these do not deal with tinnitus in the general population.

Is tinnitus a universal phenomenon?

If the definition of tinnitus is expanded to include internal sounds that are perceived in silence, tinnitus becomes an almost universal experience. In the famous experiment by Heller and Bergman (1953), subjects were asked to enter a soundproof booth and to report all the sounds they could hear. Ninety-four per cent reported some form of tinnitus-like perception. Unfortunately, there have been few attempts to replicate this finding. Graham and Newby (1962) replicated the study by Heller and Bergman (1953) but found that only 40% of their normal hearing subjects reported tinnitus. They also commented that Heller and Bergman did not assess their subjects' hearing audiometrically, which suggests that hearing impairment might have affected the outcome. In a more recent replication, Levine (2001) found that 55% of his subjects had ongoing tinnitus when they were placed in a low-noise room. Regardless of the correct figures of tinnitus in normal-hearing individuals when placed in a silent room, it is still apparent that tinnitus is a very common experience in silence, but it is often not noticed as soon as some environmental sound is present to mask that tinnitus.

Prevalence studies

A remarkably robust and comprehensive study was undertaken by the UK Medical Research Council Institute of Hearing Research and reported by Davis and El Rafaie (2000). In this study, questions about tinnitus were incorporated in a longitudinal study of hearing ($n = 48313$) and 10.1% of adults were found to have experienced prolonged (>5 minutes') spontaneous tinnitus, and in 5% of the adult population this tinnitus was reported to be moderately or severely annoying. In 0.5% tinnitus was said to have a severe effect upon the ability to lead a normal life. There is not a strict consensus on how to define tinnitus (Davis and El Rafaie, 2000), which influences interpretation of prevalence figures derived from studies conducted worldwide. An overview of some of the other published prevalence studies is given in Table 2.1. Although the definitions behind these figures are not identical, most studies have followed the five-minute criterion and have excluded temporary tinnitus. Furthermore, the response rates in the studies have varied, and there are potential biases that derive from the location of the sample. For example, Axelsson and Ringdahl (1989) studied citizens of the Swedish city of Gothenburg, whereas other studies have used nation-wide samples (Scott and Lindberg, 2000). Most studies have relied on self-reporting, which is understandable given the lack of cost-effective objective measures of tinnitus.

Table 2.1 Overview of prevalence studies

Authors	Location of study	Prevalence (%)
Hinchcliffe (1961)	Wales, Scotland	29
Leske (1981)	USA	26–44
Nagel and Drexel (1989)	Germany	11.5
Axelsson and Ringdahl (1989)	Sweden	14.2
Davis (1989)	UK	10
Parving et al. (1993)	Denmark	17
Cooper (1994)	USA	14.9
Quaranta et al. (1996)	Italy	14.5
Fabijanska et al. (1999)	Poland	5% prevalence of constant tinnitus; 20% overall
Pilgramm et al. (1999)	Germany	13
Scott and Lindberg (2000)	Sweden	15.8
Andersson et al. (2002)	Sweden	7% Internet sample; 9% postal survey
Palmer et al. (2002)	UK	6% for males and 3% for females with restriction 'most or all or the time'
Johansson and Arlinger (2003)	Sweden	13.2
Andersson et al. (Unpublished data)	Sweden	17.8

An early study by Hinchcliffe (1961) studied 800 individuals randomly recruited from two locations in the UK (Wales and Scotland). Participants were interviewed in their homes and the prevalence of tinnitus (not specifically defined) showed a tendency to increase with age from 21% (18–24 years), 27% (25–34 years), 24% (35–44 years), 27% (45–54 years), 39% (55–64 years) and 37% (65–74 years). The average was approximately 30%.

Leske (1981) reported data from a national health examination survey dating back to 1960–1962 with a total of 6672 subjects. Respondents were asked *At any time over the past few years, have you ever noticed ringing (tinnitus) in your ears or have you been bothered by other funny noises?'* Given this very broad definition, it is not surprising that as many as 32.4% of adults aged 18–79 years responded affirmatively. However, only 5.6% were said to consider tinnitus as severe, which is a figure closer to the prevalence figures of severe tinnitus usually found in other studies. Interestingly, a linear association was found between age and presence of both mild and severe tinnitus. In common with many of the following studies, a strong association was found between severity of tinnitus and hearing impairment.

In a small study with data from the German city of Ulm, Nagel and Drexel (1989) found that, of their 270 participants, 11.5% reported 'longer lasting' tinnitus, corresponding to the five-minute criterion. However, as many as

31% had noticed tinnitus at some point in time, and 19.5% had temporary tinnitus lasting not longer than five minutes. It is uncertain if this was a random sample (average cross-section), and severity of tinnitus was not clearly outlined.

Davis (1989), in a report from the National Study of Hearing, reported a tinnitus prevalence of 10%. As mentioned above, almost half of the sample studied were either moderately (2.8%) or severely (1.6%) annoyed by their tinnitus.

Axelsson and Ringdahl (1989) sent out 3600 questionnaires to a random sample of adults in the city of Gothenburg, Sweden. The response rate was 66%, and in this study tinnitus was more common in males than in females, with an overall prevalence of 14.2% for tinnitus occurring often or always.

Parving et al. (1993) studied 3387 Danish males with a median age of 63 years (range 53–75 years). A prevalence of 17% of tinnitus of more than five minutes' duration was found; 3% indicated that their tinnitus was so annoying that it interfered with sleep, reading or concentration.

Cooper (1994) reported data dating from 1971 to 1975 with 6342 subjects from the USA. Participants providing data on bothersome tinnitus ($n = 1014$) responded to the same question as used by Leske et al. (1981). Only tinnitus regarded as bothersome ('Quite a bit' or 'Just a little') was included. The overall prevalence of bothersome tinnitus was 14.9%.

Quaranta et al. (1996) studied 2170 people from the Italian cities of Bari, Florence, Milan, Padua and Palermo, with ages ranging between 18 and 80 years. Prolonged spontaneous tinnitus was found in 14.5%. The authors reported that the prevalence increased with age up to 79 years, and that manual work, dyslipidosis, hypertension, liver diseases, cervical arthrosis and alcohol consumption were statistically significant risk factors. The report was rather brief and it is uncertain to what extent participants were bothered by their tinnitus.

In a large-scale German study by Pilgramm et al. (1999) 3049 people were interviewed by telephone, which comprised 41% of the eligible people initially approached. Since this study was published as a conference proceedings report, the results were not described in much detail. The authors derived that 13% of the German population has or has once had noise in the ears lasting longer than five minutes. They also provided an estimate of those having tinnitus at the time of the investigation, which was 3.9% of the population. This latter definition is interesting, as it is a very clear definition of the presence of tinnitus. Also provided was an estimate that approximately 50% of the 3.9% of the population with ongoing tinnitus considered the effect of their tinnitus as moderately serious or unbearable. This would lead to a prevalence figure of 2% for severe tinnitus.

In a conference report on the prevalence of tinnitus in Poland, Fabijanska et al. (1999) found that, of a sample of 10349 people aged 17 years or older, 20.1% reported tinnitus (defined as lasting more than five minutes). Severe annoyance was reported by one-tenth of the tinnitus population. Increasing age was associated with increased annoyance. The authors also reported constant tinnitus, which was perceived by 4.8% of the population.

Scott and Lindberg (2000) approached a random sample of 2500 Swedish citizens from a population register (in which all citizens are registered). Responses were obtained from 1538 subjects (62%), and among these 15.8% responded 'yes' to the question, *'Have you heard buzzing, roaring or tones, or other sounds which seem to come from inside the ears or the head and that have persisted for five minutes or longer (so-called tinnitus)?'* In addition, tinnitus was graded by use of the Klockhoff and Lindblom (1967) severity definition (Scott et al., 1990) (*see* Chapter 6). As results were analysed separately for help-seeking and non-help-seeking people with tinnitus (with additional participants recruited from a clinic), no exact estimate of severe tinnitus in the general population can be derived. However, as only a minor proportion of subjects in the population survey had sought help (*n* = 7), the figures for the population-derived non-help-seeking group provide an estimate of the proportion of severe (grades II–III) tinnitus. Slightly below 50% had tinnitus of grades II–III, with only a few (12.2% of the tinnitus sample) having tinnitus of grade III. Hence, a conservative estimate is that about one person in ten has severe tinnitus in the general population.

In a prevalence study of hyperacusis, Andersson et al. (2002a) used two methods to collect data, the first being a postal survey to a random sample, of which 589 people responded (59.7% response rate). The second data collection source was the Internet, and 595 self-recruited individuals responded to a call for participants via a banner on a web page of a major Swedish newspaper home page (51.9% response rate). Also included was a question on tinnitus. The definition of tinnitus was not specified, and the assumption was made that the subjects knew what tinnitus was.

Palmer et al. (2002) studied the self-reported responses of 21201 subjects recruited from 34 general practices and members of the armed services. Ages ranged between 16 and 64 years. Questionnaire items were modelled on the National Study of Hearing (Davis, 1989). Tinnitus was defined by the question, *'During the past 12 months have you had noises in your head or ears (such as ringing, buzzing or whistling) which lasted longer than five minutes?'* One additional common restriction was that only tinnitus reported to occur most or all of the time was defined as persistent tinnitus (cf. Coles, 1984). Palmer et al. (2002) found a strong relation between self-report of tinnitus and hearing difficulties. For men, the age-standardized prevalence of persistent tinnitus was 16.1% in those who reported severe hearing difficulties, whereas for those men with slight or no hearing problems the prevalence was only 5%. For women, the corresponding figures were 33.1% and 2.6%, respectively.

In another Swedish study, Johansson and Arlinger (2003) studied 590 randomly selected subjects from the province of Östergötland in Sweden.

The prevalence of tinnitus was 13.2%, using the five minutes' definition.

Andersson et al. (unpublished data), in a recent Swedish study, made an attempt to distinguish current, 12-month and lifetime tinnitus in a random sample. The figures were 25.4% for lifetime, 21.5% for 12-month and a 17.8% point prevalence. Approximately 60% of the point prevalence group had tinnitus often or always. Annoyance was rated as average or severe in one-third of participants. In common with the findings in the National Study of Hearing (Davis and El Rafaie, 2000), only a minority reported that tinnitus had a severe effect upon their ability to lead a normal life.

It can be argued that the use of definitions to identify 'troublesome tinnitus' makes it difficult to estimate the true prevalence of tinnitus. Clearly, from a health perspective it is useful to know who is at risk of developing severe tinnitus and also the number of people who have severe tinnitus at the moment. It is apparent that the proportion of sufferers versus non-sufferers is not a static figure and, for example, publicity can influence the report of tinnitus as a significant problem (Baskill et al., 1999). This was clearly seen in Sweden in 1999 after a national campaign to raise money for tinnitus research. It should be noted, however, that many people benefit from publicity and knowing that they are not alone with their tinnitus.

Incidence

Few studies have investigated the incidence of tinnitus, that is, the number of new tinnitus cases for a predefined time period. One study by Nondahl et al. (2002) focused on tinnitus in the elderly (adults aged 48-92 years at baseline). They first sampled 3753 individuals and then returned five years later (n = 2800). The prevalence of tinnitus at baseline was 8.2%, when mild cases were excluded. The five-year incidence of new tinnitus cases was 5.7%. Interestingly, participants with tinnitus at baseline were more likely to report changing from mild tinnitus to no tinnitus (n = 135/341; 39.6%) than from mild to moderate or severe tinnitus (n = 67/341; 19.6%). The approximate incidence of 5% in older adults was also found in a Swedish longitudinal study between the ages of 70–79 years (Rubinstein et al., 1992). Pilgramm et al. (1999) estimated that, for each year, 0.33% of the German population aged over 10 become chronic tinnitus patients (with subtraction of mean mortality rate and therapy success rate). Data from the National Study of Hearing (Davis and Rafaie, 2000) indicate that 7.1% of the sample had sought the opinion of their doctor about tinnitus, and that 2.5% had attended a hospital for this purpose. Clearly, there is a need for further incidence studies.

Prevalence of tinnitus in childhood

The prevalence of tinnitus in children has been investigated and the findings are worthy of careful consideration. First, some experience of tinnitus seems to be common in childhood, and yet the problem has been underestimated (Baguley and McFerran, 1999, 2002; Davis and El Rafaie, 2000). Overall, given methodological difficulties there are few robust estimates of the prevalence of tinnitus in childhood in the general population. Nodar (1972) surveyed 2000 normally hearing children aged 11–18 years and found a tinnitus prevalence of 15%, with no further specification of annoyance. In a study by Mills et al. (1986), 93 normal-hearing children were screened for tinnitus, 29% reported tinnitus and one-third were said to be bothered by their tinnitus. Stouffer et al. (1992) used a more rigorous interview method and found that in a group of 161 children aged 7–10 years, 6% reported tinnitus, a figure that rose to 13% if less rigorous criteria were used. Holgers (2003) studied 964 school children aged 7 years. The prevalence of tinnitus in this sample was 13% among the normal-hearing children, but the possibility of priming cannot be excluded as the children were first given a lecture on hearing loss and tinnitus.

Studies have also been conducted on the prevalence of tinnitus in children with hearing impairment (Baguley and McFerran, 1999). Mills and Cherry (1984) found a prevalence of 29.5% in children with sensorineural hearing loss ($n = 66$) and 43.9% of children with ototis media ($n = 44$). In another study Mills et al. (1986) found a prevalence of 38.5% of children who were seen by otologists and said to have evidence of ear disease ($n = 267$). In one interesting study, Graham (1987) found that 66% of children with moderate or severe hearing loss reported tinnitus, whereas in children with profound hearing loss 29% did so. Druckier (1989) studied 331 children with profound hearing loss, of whom 33% reported tinnitus. Viani (1989) found a similar percentage of 23% in a sample of 102 children with severe hearing loss (aged 6–17 years). In association with a study on social competence, parents of children with hearing impairment were asked about tinnitus in their child. Only 13% were aware of any tinnitus in their child (Andersson et al., 2000a). Some researchers have argued that tinnitus in children is not annoying and that it will pass (Graham, 1981), but in a follow-up study by Martin and Snashall (1994) with 42 children with tinnitus as many as 83% still had their tinnitus at follow-up. Kentish et al. (2000) showed that children with tinnitus can suffer a great deal from their tinnitus and that they shared the problem of impaired sleep with their older adult counterparts.

The experience of tinnitus in childhood thus seems to be quite common, but it is still not clear how much these children suffer. On the basis of clinical experience and the scarce empirical data, it appears that remarkably few children are troubled by their tinnitus.

Tinnitus in old age

Tinnitus in older adults has received some interest from researchers, and it is strikingly clear that the prevalence of tinnitus increases with age. Rosenhall and Karlsson (1991) studied 674 people aged 70 years from two separate cohorts and found a prevalence of 8-15% for continuous tinnitus and 20% for occasional tinnitus. As mentioned above, Nondahl et al. (2002) found a prevalence of 8.2% in their sample of older adults. It is not easy to draw any firm conclusions from the research that has been conducted so far. For example, Hazell (1991) found that disability resulting from tinnitus did not increase with age, but this was based on clinic data and not findings from random samples. In their population-based study, Axelsson and Ringdahl (1989) found no age effect for the men, while older women experienced tinnitus as worse than younger women. This shows the importance of considering gender differences, even among the elderly. More recently, Davis and El Rafaie (2000) reported a tendency for moderate and severe annoyance to increase by age, using data from the National Study of Hearing. A similar trend can be observed in the most recent Swedish study (Andersson et al. unpublished data) as seen in Figure 2.1.

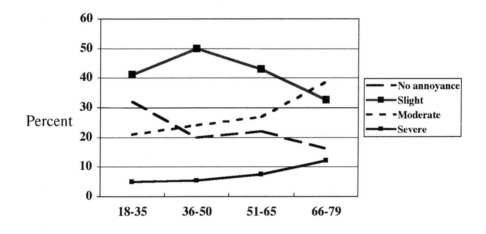

Figure 2.1 Levels of tinnitus annoyance in relation to age from Swedish population study.

Longitudinal studies

Unfortunately, there are relatively few studies on the natural history of tinnitus, and in particular the natural history of untreated tinnitus. Most of the research that has been conducted on the long-term outcome of tinnitus has been retrospective. For example, Stouffer et al. (1991) concluded that tinnitus loudness and severity increased as a function of years since onset. However, since the study was cross-sectional no definite conclusions could be drawn and the authors recommended that longitudinal studies be conducted. Smith and Coles (1987), in contrast, concluded that the severity of tinnitus was likely to decrease over time, and underscored this need in their study. This was an epidemiological study and did not focus just on clinical tinnitus. However, the data collected were retrospective. Since 25 of their subjects actually stated that tinnitus had disappeared, it is clear that tinnitus may be of a temporary nature.

Davis (1995) reported from the National Study of Hearing that, from onset to middle time, 25% of sufferers reported an increase in loudness, which was the same from middle to recent time. However, he noted that for most people loudness did not change. Data on annoyance ratings decreased for 31% of the patients from onset to middle, but the decrease was smaller (10%) from middle to recent time.

Retrospective studies of patients with vestibular schwannoma (acoustic neuroma) have been published, showing that tinnitus may arise, worsen, remain or disappear following surgery for the condition (see Chapter 4). However, this aetiology is rare and the results cannot be extrapolated to individuals with the more common causes of tinnitus, such as noise-induced hearing loss. More is known about the natural history of tinnitus in the elderly. Rubinstein et al. (1992) found substantial longitudinal fluctuations in tinnitus and a high occurrence of spontaneous remission. Patients were studied at the ages of 70, 75 and 79 years, and results showed that tinnitus had increased in severity in 25% of the women, and decreased in 58%, leaving 17% unchanged. For the men, tinnitus increased in 8% and decreased in 39%, with a larger proportion unchanged (53%). Although the long term outcome of tinnitus in Ménière's disease has been studied (Green et al. 1991), gradings of tinnitus severity have seldom been reported, vertigo being the symptom drawing most attention. In a longitudinal study, data were collected for an average period of five years post treatment in a sample of tinnitus patients who had received cognitive behavioural therapy (Andersson et al., 2001). Results showed decreases in annoyance and an increase in tolerance of tinnitus. Maskability of tinnitus at the commencement of treatment was a predictor of tinnitus-related distress at follow-up. Folmer (2002) studied 190 patients who returned follow-up questionnaires, on average, 22 months after their initial tinnitus clinic appointment. The group exhibited significant decreases of tinnitus distress, depression and anxiety.

Localization of tinnitus

Numerous studies have reported the site of tinnitus, and a common observation is that tinnitus most commonly is bilateral (at least 50%), followed by unilateral on the left side and then unilateral on the right side. There are other cases in which tinnitus is localized in the head, and a few cases in which tinnitus is perceived as an external sound. The observation that tinnitus is more common on the left side is interesting. One possible cause for this asymmetry could be that hearing loss is more common in the left ear. However, Meikle and Greist (1992) found that noise exposure in the left ear (for example, by gun shooting) could not explain the difference. Another potential cause could be neural imbalance at a cortical level, and indeed Min and Lee (1997) noted that somatic symptoms overall tend to be lateralized to the left rather than to the right. There is no clear evidence that left-sided tinnitus is more annoying than right-sided tinnitus, nor that it is associated with greater degrees of hearing loss (Cahani et al., 1984; Budd et al., 1995). Tyler (1997) questioned if there are true cases of unilateral tinnitus. First, the auditory pathway has many cross pathways, and second, patients with supposedly unilateral tinnitus may report tinnitus on the previously unaffected side when the contralateral tinnitus is masked. However, Tyler (1997) concluded that it is common for tinnitus to be dominant in one ear, but that does not prove that tinnitus originates from that ear. Davis and El Rafaie (2000) suggested that the concept of left versus right ear differences needs more detailed research studies. Interestingly, Erlandsson et al. (1992) found that multiple localizations of tinnitus were associated with more distress, again a finding that merits further investigation.

Seeking help

It is far from the case that all people with tinnitus seek any help. Davis (1995) reported that despite the frequency of the symptom in the population, only 7% of the population had consulted any doctor for their tinnitus and only 2.5% had sought specialist advice from an otologist. In a Swedish study, 13% of the respondents with tinnitus had been to a physician for tinnitus during the past 12 months (Andersson et al., unpublished data).

Summary

Prevalence studies suggest that tinnitus is a common problem in the general population of many first-world countries, with an approximate prevalence of 10–15%. There is a dearth of information about tinnitus in the developing countries. The majority of people who experience prolonged spontaneous tinnitus are not severely distressed by the symptom, but tinnitus does constitute a significant problem for 0.5–3% of the population. The natural history of tinnitus is only partly known, but there are indications that the perception of tinnitus generally becomes less annoying over time. Tinnitus experience is common among children, but the mechanisms and natural history of tinnitus in children remain unknown to a large extent. Older people often have tinnitus, and studies suggest that their tinnitus is perceived as particularly annoying. The incidence of tinnitus is not known, apart from a 5% estimate for a five-year period. Tinnitus localization is well known, but there are no strong explanations for why tinnitus is more prevalent in the left ear.

Characterization of annoyance in relation to tinnitus is not clearly defined in behavioural terms. Most studies to date have used questionnaire assessment. In contrast, major studies on psychiatric disturbances commonly use structured interviews, which could be an alternative in future epidemiological work on tinnitus.

Chapter 3
Mechanisms

Many cases of tinnitus seen clinically are associated with otological pathologies, encompassing the whole gamut of ear disease – from the sudden sensorineural hearing loss after a temporal bone fracture to the gradual onset of deafness in presbyacusis. Consequently, much effort has been put into trying to understand the pathophysiological events by which these otological conditions give rise to tinnitus. However, there are other forms of tinnitus in which there is no obvious otological trigger: sudden emotional stimulation in the form of a major life event such as bereavement, illness or psychological shock can precipitate the onset of tinnitus. Similarly, many cases of tinnitus arise without otological or emotional change. There is also an interesting sub-group of tinnitus patients whose trigger factors appear to arise in other sensory systems. Even if there is an otological trigger, there is good evidence that the tinnitus activity can occur at an anatomical site distant to the initial pathology. For example, tinnitus associated with a vestibular schwannoma often continues after surgical excision of the triggering lesion. Therefore it has become apparent to the scientific community that concentrating on the pathological event that triggered the tinnitus may not be very helpful in managing the condition. Nevertheless it is still useful to examine the various suggested triggering mechanisms, as, by understanding specific cases, more general understanding may follow.

Tinnitus mechanisms associated with the cochlea

Discordant damage of inner and outer hair cells

Noise and ototoxic agents, such as aminoglycoside antibiotics, typically cause maximal hearing loss in the 4 kHz to 6 kHz range. This corresponds with an area of hair cell damage in the basal turn of the cochlea, and outer hair cells have been demonstrated to be more susceptible to damage than inner hair cells (Stypulkowski, 1990). In the area of maximum damage both inner and outer hair cell cilia are destroyed. However, at the junction between damaged cochlea and normal cochlea there is an area where the outer hair cell cilia are destroyed but the inner hair cell cilia remain. Jastreboff (1990, 1995) suggested that this would result in imbalanced activity between the Type I nerve fibres that synapse with the inner hair cells and the Type II fibres that synapse with the outer hair cells. This results in imbalanced activity further up the auditory pathways, possibly in the dorsal cochlear nucleus, which in turn causes change at higher centres that may be perceived as tinnitus. In the normal cochlea the tectorial membrane touches the tips of the outer hair cell cilia but does not touch the inner hair cell cilia. It has been suggested that in a damaged cochlea, at the region where inner hair cell cilia are still present but outer hair cell cilia are missing the tectorial membrane sags down on to the inner hair cell cilia causing them to depolarize. There is clinical evidence to support this theory: some patients with high-frequency sensorineural hearing loss have tinnitus that corresponds in pitch with the frequency at which the hearing loss begins (Hazell, 1987; Hazell and Jastreboff, 1990). Jastreboff (1995) refined this hypothesis by suggesting that the brain might try to overcome what it saw as dysfunctional outer hair cells by increasing efferent neural activity to those outer hair cells. Clearly, without functioning outer hair cells this efferent activity would be futile within the cochlea but it is possible that it might alter the central perception of inner hair cell input, causing an apparent increase in activity.

Discordant damage in normal hearing

It is possible to damage quite a large proportion of outer hair cells – perhaps as many as 30% – without causing a measurable hearing loss by use of standard audiometric techniques (Clark et al., 1984). Thus, in areas of the cochlea where there are missing outer hair cell cilia there may be increased activity in inner hair cells and therefore an increase in neural activity in Type I nerve fibres carrying auditory information to the brain.

Discordant damage in profound hearing loss

If damage to both inner hair cells and outer hair cells is uniform there will be no imbalance in neural activity. Thus, a cochlea that has lost all or most of both populations of hair cells may not generate the central neural activity that is perceived as tinnitus. The clinical observation that 30% of people with profound sensorineural hearing loss do not have tinnitus (Hazell, 1996) supports this theory.

Otoacoustic emissions

Otoacoustic emissions are small sounds generated by the ear. They originate from mechanical activity in the outer hair cells of the cochlea and are then transmitted through the endolymph, oval window, ossicular chain and tympanic membrane. Otoacoustic emissions can be spontaneous or can arise in response to sound input to the ear, in which case they are known as 'evoked otoacoustic emissions'. Although it had been suggested as early as 1948 by Gold that ears could produce sound, this initial suggestion was that such sound was generated as a result of biomechanical imperfections in the auditory system. This remained a hypothesis until 1978, when Kemp described a means of measuring sound generated by the ear and went on to suggest that these sounds were generated as a normal otological function rather than a defect.

There was much initial excitement in the tinnitus field, with the hope that people who had tinnitus would have spontaneous otoacoustic emissions corresponding to their tinnitus. This hope was rapidly dashed: various studies showed that 38–60% of adults with normal hearing have spontaneous otoacoustic emissions (Hall, 2000). The majority of these people are unaware of this activity (Wilson and Sutton, 1981). Further work by Penner and Burns (1987) showed that even if a patient has tinnitus and spontaneous otoacoustic emissions, the perceived frequency of the tinnitus rarely matches that of the spontaneous otoacoustic emissions. Various studies have shown that only between 2% and 4.5% of tinnitus patients have tinnitus that can be ascribed to spontaneous otoacoustic emissions. Additionally, Long and Tubis (1988) showed that if tinnitus is a manifestation of spontaneous otoacoustic emissions activity, abolition of the spontaneous otoacoustic emissions would be expected to reduce or abolish the tinnitus. There is only one reported case in which aspirin has abolished spontaneous otoacoustic emissions-associated tinnitus (Penner and Coles, 1992), and this procedure entails risk to hearing and exacerbated tinnitus.

Calcium

Calcium transport is an important factor in the normal functioning of the cochlea. The stereocilia of inner hair cells and outer hair cells are surrounded by endolymph, which is a high-potassium, low-sodium fluid. The base of each hair cell is surrounded by perilymph, which is a low-potassium, high-sodium, high-calcium solution. Incoming sound sets up waveforms in the basilar membrane which displaces the hair cell stereocilia from their resting position. This mechanical change results in the opening of ion channels on the stereocilia. Ashmore and Gale (2000) suggested that these channels are like tiny lids at the base of the tip link structures that run between adjacent stereocilia (Figure 3.1).

The opening of these channels allows potassium to pour into the hair cells, changing the electrical potential and thereby causing voltage-gated calcium channels to open. In inner hair cells this results in neurotransmitter release, which in turn attaches to receptors on nerve fibres and, when enough receptors have been activated, produces an action potential in the auditory nerve (Wangemann and Schact, 1996). In outer hair cells the

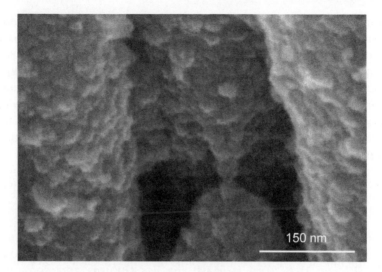

Figure 3.1 Scanning electron micrograph of a close-up of the stereocilia, showing a tip link connecting the shorter stereocilium in front with the taller stereocilium behind. (Micrograph supplied by DN Furness, Keele University.)

opening of the calcium channels results in the slow motility response (Holley, 1996). The calcium that has entered the hair cells is then buffered by intracellular polypeptides, sequestered in the endoplasmic reticulum and finally returned to the perilymph via an active membrane pump which is under the control of calmodulin (Blaustein, 1988), a second messenger protein. Calcium flux is also implicated in the electrical repolarization of the hair cell.

Because calcium is so fundamental to the normal physiology of the hair cells, there have been various suggestions that defects in calcium handling could be implicated in cochlear malfunction (Zenner and Ernst, 1993). In 1990 Jastreboff suggested several mechanisms by which this might result in tinnitus. Prominent among these suggestions was the hypothesis that calcium concentrations might directly affect neurotransmitter release. Raised levels initially increase auditory nerve activity in response to mechanical stimulation of the cochlea while reducing spontaneous activity. Further increase causes reduction of both evoked and spontaneous activity. Reduction of calcium concentration conversely causes reduced evoked activity and increased spontaneous activity. Jastreboff (1990) suggested that reduced extracellular calcium concentration could alter the signal to noise ratio by increasing spontaneous activity and reducing evoked activity, increasing the likelihood of developing tinnitus.

Both salicylates and quinine cause a rise in intracellular calcium that would be expected to have the same effect as reducing extracellular calcium. An animal model of tinnitus was developed by Jastreboff et al. (1988) by conditioning male pigmented rats to suppress licking when exposed to sound. Administration of quinine in ototoxic concentrations (Jastreboff et al., 1991) produced the same lick suppression as external sound. Further experiments showed that the rats' response to quinine- and salicylate-induced 'tinnitus' could be abolished by administration of calcium or nimodipine, which blocks the voltage-gated calcium channels (Penner and Jastreboff, 1996).

N-methyl-D-aspartate receptors

Stress is well recognized as being important in both the emergence and maintenance of tinnitus in many individuals. Although it has been generally thought that this is a purely central effect there are suggestions that stress may have a peripheral role too. Glutamate is an excitatory neurotransmitter released by inner hair cells in response to mechanical stimulation (Puel, 1995). This transmitter interacts with several receptors on Type 1 auditory fibres, including N-methyl-D-aspartate receptors (NMDA). Dynorphins are endogenous peptides that function as selective agonists for kappa opioid receptors. Dynorphins are released into the synaptic regions between inner hair cells and Type 1 auditory fibres by lateral efferent neurons in response to stressful situations. Sahley and Nodar (2001) suggested that dynorphins could potentiate the effect of glutamate on the NMDA receptors and postulated that chronic exposure could result in abnormal excitement in the auditory nerve.

An animal model has been produced that suggests that salicylates give rise to tinnitus by activating NMDA receptors (Guitton et al., 2003). Rats were conditioned to perform a motor task in response to sound. Both salicylate and mefenamate, a non-steroidal anti-inflammatory compound, interfered with the rats' ability to perform their task: the number of correct responses fell but the number of false positive responses in which the rats performed their task in the absence of noise rose. This was interpreted as showing that the drugs had induced tinnitus in the rats. Salicylate inhibits the enzyme cyclo-oxygenase, which prevents production of prostaglandins but causes a rise in precursor chemicals such as arachidonic acid. Arachidonic acid is known to potentiate NMDA channels so the experiment was repeated with an antagonist of NMDA receptors instilled into the perilymph. This blocked the rise in false positive responses, supporting the hypothesis that salicylates induce tinnitus by indirectly stimulating NMDA receptors.

Retrocochlear tinnitus

Theories of altered neural activity

There is always some background and stochastic electrical activity in the auditory nerve even if there is no sound input to the ear. Initial theories of tinnitus generation were based on the hypothesis that tinnitus was caused by increase of this spontaneous activity (Evans et al., 1981). However, there was conflicting experimental evidence as to whether cochlear dysfunction caused an increase or decrease in this spontaneous neural activity. Kiang et al. (1970) studied cats that had received the ototoxic antibiotic kanamycin and discovered reduced spontaneous activity in the cochlear nerve. Evans et al. (1981) studied cats that had received salicylate at a dosage equivalent to that known to cause tinnitus in humans (400 mg/kg). They demonstrated that the cats had developed a hearing loss and found an increase in spontaneous activity in the auditory nerve. At a lower dosage of 200 mg/kg this effect was not seen. Tyler (1984) pointed out methodological differences between these two studies and indicated that recordings from single units of the cochlear nerve might be misrepresentative of the whole nerve. Eggermont (2000) also considered these findings and suggested that, even if such animal experiments could be extrapolated to humans, it was unlikely that changes in spontaneous activity in the VIIIth nerve were implicated in human tinnitus experiences.

There is also spontaneous neural activity within the central auditory pathways. There have been various reports showing that intense sound exposure increases the spontaneous activity in the dorsal cochlear nucleus of the golden hamster (Kaltenbach and McAslin, 1996; Kaltenbach et al., 1996; Kaltenbach et al., 1999). Similar experiments on chinchillas showed increased spontaneous activity in both the inferior colliculus and dorsal cochlear nucleus (Salvi et al., 1996). There was also tonotopic reorganization in these structures. Chen et al. (1999) exposed rats to intense sound and recorded spontaneous activity in the dorsal cochlear nucleus. Although there was an increase in bursting activity there was a reduction of regular, simple spiking activity, suggesting a possible increase in auditory efferent activity.

Ototoxic agents such as salicylate (aspirin) were shown to produce increased spontaneous activity in the inferior colliculus of both rats (Chen and Jastreboff, 1995) and guinea-pigs (Jastreboff and Sasaki, 1986). Increased spontaneous activity in the cortex of gerbils after noise exposure or salicylate administration has been demonstrated using 2-deoxyglucose techniques (Wallhäusser-Franke et al., 1996) and c-fos immunochemistry (Wallhäusser-Franke, 1997). Wallhäusser-Franke and Langner (1999) demonstrated increased spontaneous activity in the amygdalae of such animals and postulated that this might represent a limbic response to tinnitus, though they could not exclude other forms of stress as the cause. Langner and Wallhäusser-Franke (1999) went on to present a computer model of tinnitus based on these results. Salicylate administration does not cause increased activity in the ventral cochlear nucleus, suggesting that the drug's effects are not caused by increased afferent activity in the cochlear nerve (Zhang and Kaltenbach, 1998).

Medial efferent system

Eggermont (2000) used the observation that tinnitus is often worsened by stress and can be alleviated by biofeedback techniques to propose that the medial efferent system might play a role in tinnitus perception. The efferent system is closely linked to the reticular formation in the brainstem, and Hazell and Jastreboff (1990) suggested that such links would help to explain how tinnitus produces its alerting effect. Jastreboff and Hazell (1993) also suggested that the efferent system might be able to modify pre-existing cochlear tinnitus. However, experimental evidence for efferent system implication in tinnitus is not strong. Veuillet et al. (1992) performed an experiment that measured transient evoked otoacoustic emissions in patients with unilateral tinnitus while noise was applied to the contralateral ear. They hypothesized that efferent dysfunction would cause less transient evoked otoacoustic emission suppression in the tinnitus ear compared with the non-tinnitus ear. The hypothesis was weakly supported by the results, but there was marked inter-subject variability. A similar experiment by Lind (1996) showed no statistical difference between the ears. Baguley et al. (2002) reviewed vestibular nerve section in humans. Efferent auditory information runs in the inferior vestibular nerve and therefore section of the nerve would be expected to modify tinnitus. This was not the case.

Somatic modulation

It has been recognized for a considerable time that a small number of patients are able to modify their tinnitus by performing somatic tasks, such as clenching their jaws (Lockwood et al., 1998) or stimulating their skin (Cacace et al., 1999a, 1999b). In 1999 Levine investigated this phenomenon by asking all patients attending the tinnitus clinic to perform a series of head and neck contractions. Over two-thirds (68%) reported a change in their tinnitus: loudness, pitch and laterality could all be affected. Decrease in tinnitus was more likely to occur if the tinnitus was unilateral. Some of the patients were also asked to perform extremity contractions. These were less likely to affect the tinnitus. The findings were used to suggest that somatic inputs could disinhibit the ipsilateral dorsal cochlear nucleus, acting via the medullary somatosensory nucleus. This disinhibition could affect spontaneous activity in the dorsal cochlear nucleus, altering tinnitus perception. Connections between the dorsal cochlear nucleus and medullary somatosensory nucleus have been identified in cats and are thought to be important in relating pinna location and sound localization (Nelken and Young, 1996). The anatomical evidence in humans is, however, less clear. Levine (1999) went on to speculate that somatic modulation is a fundamental property of tinnitus.

Analogies with pain

Tinnitus has long been compared to pain. Both conditions can follow a variety of different peripheral pathologies, both can be governed by different mechanisms, both are highly subjective and both are difficult to treat. Also, like tinnitus, chronic pain can be a sequel to a peripheral injury even after the peripheral injury has resolved. Møller (1997) concluded that both chronic pain and tinnitus are caused by central nervous system changes and that the site of this change is not the same as the perceived site of the problem. Different types of pain respond to different types of treatment. Møller (1997) suggested that there may be specific forms of tinnitus that may have specific solutions and that to amass all forms of tinnitus and base treatment strategies accordingly may be misleading.

Phantom limb pain is a specific entity that seems to have strong similarities to tinnitus. Cortical reorganization is thought to be the explanation for phantom limb pain, and several workers have suggested that a similar process applies to tinnitus (Salvi et al., 2000). Central auditory pathways normally display precise tonotopicity. If part of the cochlea is damaged, a corresponding part of the auditory cortex becomes deafferented. The deafferented cortex has the same characteristic frequency as the damaged cochlea and the immediate effect is that neuronal activity in that area is reduced (Robertson and Irvine, 1989). Several months later neuronal activity has returned to the deafferented cortex but now the neurones have the characteristic frequencies of the adjacent undamaged cochlea (Harrison et al., 1991). This results in the frequencies represented at the upper and lower edges of the damaged area being over-represented centrally. Salvi et al. (2000) suggested that the increased activity in these areas of the cortex could be interpreted as tinnitus. This could be another mechanism to explain the observation (Jastreboff and Hazell, 1993) that the pitch of tinnitus is often perceived at the margin of an area of cochlear damage. Although reorganization is thought to be primarily a cortical phenomenon it has also been described in the inferior colliculus (Salvi et al., 2000).

Gaze-evoked tinnitus

Gaze-evoked tinnitus is a condition in which tinnitus can be modified by altering the direction of gaze from a neutral position. It was originally recognized as a rare sequel to surgery for cerebellopontine angle tumours (Whittaker, 1982). The phenomenon has now been recognized as being more common than previously thought (Giraud et al., 1999; Biggs and Ramsden, 2002) and various suggestions have been promoted to explain the condition. As it seems to follow deafferentation, most theories have focused on central neural plasticity. It has been suggested that cross-modal neurons sprout to occupy synapses that have been denervated, previously silent synapses become unmasked or ephaptic interactions occur (Wall et al., 1987; Cacace et al., 1994).

Ephaptic coupling

Ephaptic coupling is a process in which a cell membrane can become excited because it comes into contact with an adjacent cell membrane that is already excited. Impulses are normally passed along the auditory nerve fibres without exciting adjacent fibres, electrical transmission generally occurring only at synapses. However, in certain circumstances this insulation effect can fail, allowing signals to spread throughout the nerve – causing cross-talk. This phenomenon has been implicated in hemifacial spasm and trigeminal neuralgia (Møller, 1984). Blood vessels pressing against the facial and trigeminal nerves, respectively, are thought to be responsible for these conditions in some instances, and surgical separation of the vessels has been reported to control the symptoms successfully. Møller (1984) suggested that this could apply to the VIIIth cranial nerve too, and pressure from blood vessels or tumours such as vestibular schwannomas could increase neural activity within the nerve, which might be perceived as tinnitus. Eggermont (1990) suggested that a space-occupying lesion, such as a vestibular schwannoma, would cause breakdown of the myelin sheath of the auditory nerve, resulting in tinnitus.

Stochastic resonance

Stochastic resonance is a phenomenon in which a signal within a system is too weak for the system to detect. However, in certain circumstances it is possible for this weak signal to resonate with noise in the system – producing enhancement and thereby enabling detection of the signal. Several animal senses use this technique as a means of detecting sensory inputs that would otherwise be too small to notice. It has been suggested that this process could also enhance the spontaneous pseudo-random firing within the auditory nerve, resulting in tinnitus (Baguley, 1997).

5HT

5HT (5 hydroxytryptamine), or serotonin, is an amine produced by the hydroxylation and decarboxylation of the essential amino acid tryptophan. Receptors are found mainly in the gut and brain, and exist in many forms. 5HT receptors are found in the auditory nuclei of the brainstem (Thompson et al., 1994). Increased levels of 5HT in the central nervous system generally have an inhibitory effect and have been shown to reduce the auditory startle reflex (Davis et al., 1980). Thus, reduced levels of 5HT might be expected to have an excitatory effect in the central auditory pathways and this has been suggested as a cause of both tinnitus (Simpson and Davies, 2000) and hyperacusis (Marriage and Barnes, 1995). However, to date, drugs that increase 5HT concentrations, such as monoamine oxidase inhibitors and selective serotonin reuptake inhibitors, have not proved beneficial.

Summary

The experimental evidence supports the theory that there are multiple possible mechanisms for tinnitus generation, occurring at all levels of the auditory pathways. This diversity of causation of this single symptom may help to explain why no 'cure-all' for tinnitus has yet been discovered. In many cases it may be more accurate to talk about *association* with tinnitus onset, rather than direct causality. In current clinical practice, treatment strategies are largely based on either Jastreboff's neurophysiological model or the psychological model. They address the distress that tinnitus generates rather than treat the underlying cause of the symptom. As knowledge of the pathophysiology of the condition improves it is hoped that more precise therapeutic tools will become available.

Chapter 4
Medical models of tinnitus

Research into tinnitus is hindered by the fact that tinnitus patients display marked heterogeneity. Although most patients with tinnitus have no more serious otological pathology than cochlear degeneration appropriate to their age and previous noise exposure, there are a few specific diseases that incorporate tinnitus as a key symptom. Such cases of tinnitus, sometimes referred to as 'syndromic tinnitus', have received much interest in a hope that understanding a few highly defined examples of tinnitus would clarify the greater picture. Similarly, there are a few drugs that induce tinnitus and much effort has been directed towards understanding the route by which this occurs.

Drug-induced tinnitus

Even a casual perusal of drug data sheets reveals that many have tinnitus listed as a potential side effect. Some have direct effects on the cochlea, some may act on receptors in the central auditory pathways, but in many cases the mode of action is unknown. In addition there are some less obvious routes by which drugs are involved in tinnitus: drugs are given in response to health-related problems, and both the problem that requires the treatment and the treatment itself are potent stimulants of the limbic system. This limbic system activation could account for onset of tinnitus rather than direct effects of the drug.

Commonly reported drugs causing tinnitus include salicylates and some of the other non-steroidal anti-inflammatory drugs (NSAIDs); certain antibiotics such as the aminoglycosides and ciprofloxacin; quinine and other similar antimalarial agents; loop diuretics such as furosemide; and cytotoxic agents such as cisplatin. The mechanisms of tinnitus generation are best understood for salicylates and aminoglycosides.

Salicylates generally have a reversible, dose-related ototoxic effect, although permanent effects have been reported (Miller, 1985). Mammano and Ashmore (1993) reported that salicylates affect the outer hair cells, decoupling stereocilia from the tectorial membrane. Acetyl salicylic acid (aspirin) has been shown to abolish spontaneous otoacoustic emissions (McFadden and Pasanen, 1994) adding clinical evidence that salicylates cause outer hair cell dysfunction. Jung et al. (1993) demonstrated that salicylates reduce cochlear blood flow, but as the endolymph potential remains unchanged with aspirin administration it is unlikely that reduced perfusion in the stria vascularis is very important in salicylate-induced tinnitus (Puel et al., 1990). Salicylates inhibit the enzyme cyclo-oxygenase (also known as 'prostaglandin synthetase') thereby reducing prostaglandin production and reducing inflammation. However, some of the arachidonic acid that was to be turned into prostaglandins under the control of cyclo-oxygenase is then diverted into leukotriene production. It has been suggested that leukotrienes are implicated in tinnitus generation (Jung et al., 1997).

Aminoglycoside antibiotics such as gentamicin have their antimicrobial action by acting on ribosomes and preventing polypeptide synthesis. The parentrally administered aminoglycosides have maximal effect on bacterial ribosomes and relatively little effect on mammalian ribosomes. However, if the concentration of aminoglycosides exceeds normal therapeutic limits ototoxicity can occur, and in 1981 Bernard demonstrated histopathological evidence of outer hair cell damage in cats that had been treated with gentamicin. There are certain human families that display unusually high cochlear sensitivity to aminoglycosides. Investigation of these families has shown a mutation of a mitochondrial gene, small ribosomal RNA gene (12S rRNA) (Prezant et al., 1993; Cortopassi and Hutchin, 1994). Like all mitochondrial genes, this is passed down the maternal line. Outer hair cells have high metabolic requirements and consequently have high concentrations of mitochondria. The altered gene makes the mitochondria and hence the outer hair cells more susceptible to aminoglycoside damage.

Many of the drugs that have a specific ototoxic effect, such as the aminoglycoside antibiotics and cytotoxic agents, are given only for life-threatening conditions and their usage is often unavoidable. To minimize the risk of ototoxicity, plasma levels of the drug should be monitored to keep the drug level within its therapeutic range. Identifying particularly susceptible individuals should also help to limit iatrogenic tinnitus.

Although there have been anecdotal reports of recreational drugs such as cannabis and ecstasy either causing or relieving tinnitus, there is no good evidence to support either argument. Studies on the effect of cannabis on hearing suggest that the drug has little effect on the auditory system (Liedgren et al., 1976). The case with alcohol is also confused: there have been suggestions that alcohol in large quantities can damage the cochlea (Quick, 1973) or adversely affect central auditory pathways (Spitzer and Ventry, 1980). Despite these findings, reports on the effect of alcohol on tinnitus have shown both exacerbation and relief of the symptom (Ronis, 1984; Pugh et al., 1995).

Otosclerosis

Otosclerosis is a disease of the bone of the otic capsule, which is the bone that forms the cochlea, vestibular apparatus and the footplate of the stapes.

Clinically, patients present with conductive hearing loss that may start as a unilateral loss but usually eventually affects both ears. The patients may display paracusis Willisi (better hearing in noisy environment). Later in the disease sensorineural loss may occur. Tinnitus is present in the majority and occasionally is the presenting symptom. In the early stages of otosclerosis the tinnitus may have a pulsatile nature. Later, as the disease progresses and sensorineural hearing loss supervenes, the tinnitus tends to be non-pulsatile. Vertigo is present in 25% of patients with otosclerosis. The tympanic membranes usually look normal, though a red flush may be apparent. This finding is referred to as 'Schwartze's sign' and is indicative of active disease. Audiology typically shows a hearing loss with an air–bone gap and a dip in bone conduction at 2 kHz called the 'Carhart notch'. There is reduced compliance on tympanometry and reduced or absent stapedial reflex. High resolution CT scanning shows thickening of otic capsule bone with surrounding rarefaction. Estimates of the prevalence of otosclerosis vary from 0.3% (Morrison and Bundey, 1970) to 2.1% of the adult population (Browning and Gatehouse, 1992). The annual incidence of otosclerosis in Sweden was reported as 12 per 100 000 in 1973 (Stahle et al., 1978) and 6.1 per 100 000 in 1981 (Levin et al., 1988). Clinical otosclerosis is more common in women by a ratio of 2:1. It is more common in caucasians compared with negros by a ratio of 10:1. Onset is generally between the ages of 11 and 40 years, and the condition tends to progress in puberty and pregnancy. There have also been suggestions that administered female sex hormones, such as hormone replacement therapy (HRT), can cause progression of otosclerosis – though this is still disputed. Histological evidence of otosclerosis is much more common than clinical otosclerosis and there is no sex incidence variation with histological otosclerosis.

The aetiology of otosclerosis remains incompletely understood. There is often a positive family history and the condition does seem to have a genetic basis in 50–70% of cases (Levin et al., 1988). The mode of inheritance in these cases seems to be autosomal dominant with variable penetration. Arnold and Friedmann (1988) suggested that previous measles infection played a role. Other hypotheses include metabolic, immune, vascular and traumatic aetiologies.

There are several theories as to how otosclerosis causes tinnitus:

- conductive hearing losses reduce the masking effect of environmental sound
- the new bone formed has a rich blood supply, causing pulsatile tinnitus (Gibson, 1973)
- the otosclerotic process produces small arteriovenous malformations (abnormal connections between arteries and veins) resulting in pulsatile tinnitus (Sismanis and Smoker, 1994)
- cochlear tinnitus caused by: toxic enzymes produced by the otosclerotic bone damage the cochlea; bony invasion of the cochlea; damage to the cochlear blood supply.

In the early twentieth century it was recognized that the hearing loss of otosclerosis had a mechanical cause and was potentially amenable to surgery. Modern microsurgical apparatus and techniques were not available and therefore surgery on the ossicles was not feasible. In the 1920s the operation of fenestration was developed and later popularized by Lempert (1938). This involved performing a mastoidectomy and then removing some of the bone over the membranous labyrinth. This allowed sound to bypass the conductive block and pass straight into the inner ear. This improved the hearing but did not return it to normal. Also, the operation produced a large mastoid cavity with all its attendant disadvantages and patients often suffered from dizziness post-operatively. Once microsurgical techniques had been developed further therapeutic options became possible, and in 1952 the operation of stapes mobilization was developed by Rosen. He noticed that if one gently pressed the stapes of someone with otosclerosis, the hearing often improved – albeit temporarily. The operation worked by breaking the bony union between the stapes footplate and the round window. Unfortunately, the otosclerotic process usually began again and the stapes became fused with the round window once more. In 1958 Shea developed the operation of stapedectomy, in which the stapes is removed and replaced with a prosthesis. Initially, the whole stapes bone was removed; now, most surgeons remove only the superstructure and then make a small hole, or fenestra, through the footplate with micro-instruments, a micro-drill or laser.

Current treatment options include:
- observation
- hearing aid amplification
- sodium fluoride, 50 mg daily for two years (this should be avoided in children, pregnant women, patients with rheumatoid arthritis and patients with renal disease)
- stapedectomy.

Several studies have looked at tinnitus following stapedectomy operations. Gersdorff et al. (2000) found disappearance of tinnitus in 64%, improvement in 16%, no change in 14% and worsening in 6%. Surprisingly, the outcome with respect to the tinnitus was unrelated to the hearing outcome. Ayache et al. (2003) studied 62 patients undergoing stapes surgery for otosclerosis. Pre-operative tinnitus was present in 74%. Among these patients the tinnitus ceased in 55.9%, reduced in 32.4%, remained unchanged in 8.8% and worsened in 2.9%. Among the patients who did not have pre-operative tinnitus, none developed tinnitus in the immediate post-operative period. Surgical technique has been investigated with reference to tinnitus outcome: modern small fenestra surgical techniques gave a better outcome than operations in which the footplate was removed (Gersdorff et al., 2000).

Other forms of conductive hearing loss

Conditions such as impacted wax, glue ear (secretory otitis media, otitis media with effusion), perforations of the tympanic membrane or cholesteatoma (chronic otitis media, chronic suppurative otitis media) can all be associated with tinnitus. These are all common conditions: the prevalence of chronic otitis media in the UK is estimated at 4.1% (Browning and Gatehouse, 1992).

In 1984, Mills and Cherry reported a series of 66 children (aged 5–15 years) who presented to an ENT outpatient clinic with otitis media with effusion. Of these children, 29 (43.9%) reported tinnitus when asked. Forty-four children with sensorineural hearing loss were chosen as a control group: there was no use of a normally hearing control group. Among the sensorineural hearing loss control subjects 13 (29.5%) reported tinnitus.

Much of the tinnitus perception in conductive hearing loss is probably due to reduction of environmental sound input, allowing better perception of sensorineural tinnitus or somatosounds. Additionally, central gain in the auditory system may increase in the presence of a conductive lesion. Some tinnitus in chronic suppurative otitis media may be iatrogenic, a consequence of using ototoxic ear drops. Theoretically, the group of patients with conductive lesions should be relatively easily treated. Wax can be removed, glue can be aspirated, grommets can be inserted, perforations can be repaired and ossicles can be reconstructed or replaced. However, if the operation is being performed specifically for tinnitus these patients need very careful counselling before undertaking surgery. Surgery is a profound stimulant of the limbic system and hence tends to increase tinnitus peri-operatively. Also, tympanomastoid surgery usually increases any conductive loss in the immediate post-operative period because of swelling and haematoma in the middle ear and dressing packs in the ear canal. Patients need to be warned to expect this. Lastly, there is always a risk with middle ear surgery that the inner ear will be damaged inadvertently.

Although conductive hearing loss is common, and tinnitus is common in conductive hearing loss, there is a dearth of good trials on the effect of surgery upon any tinnitus in these patients. Helms (1981) looked at the effects of tympanoplasty on patients with perforations of the tympanic membrane associated with tinnitus. Approximately one-third had less tinnitus post-operatively, one-third were unchanged and one-third were worse.

Ménière's disease

In 1861 Prosper Ménière described an otological disease that subsequently became eponymous. In the classical form of Ménière's disease the clinical picture is easy to recognize: episodic attacks with prodromal aural fullness and tinnitus followed by acute vertigo and hearing loss. The episodes tend to last for a period of hours and the patient then recovers. The hearing loss is characteristically maximal at low frequencies and with recurrent attacks tends to become permanent rather than temporary. Estimating the prevalence of the condition is fraught because the diagnostic criteria for Ménière's disease were originally rather loose: a study in the UK suggested a disease occurence of 157 per 100 000 (Cawthorne and Hewlett, 1954). In an attempt to facilitate accurate research on the condition, the American Academy of Otolaryngology – Head and Neck Surgery (Committee on Hearing and Equilibrium, 1995) created a set of criteria for making a diagnosis of Ménière's disease. Observing these criteria, a survey in Finland showed a disease prevalence of 43 per 100 000 with an annual incidence of up to 4.3 per 100 000 (Kotimaki et al., 1999).

In 1938, Hallpike and Cairns described the histopathological findings in Ménière's disease with dilatation of the scala media and saccule, suggesting that excessive endolymph, or endolymphatic hydrops, was the cause of the condition. It subsequently became apparent that endolymphatic hydrops was a pathological condition seen in several other conditions as well as Ménière's disease (Table 4.1).

By definition, Ménière's disease is primary endolymphatic hydrops and various theories have been suggested for the pathogenesis of the disease (Gibson and Arenberg, 1997):

- congenital predisposition
- defects of endolymph production or absorption
- local hormones (saccin) and hydrophyllic proteins
- systemic hormones (vasopressin)
- autoimmunity
- allergy

Just as there is dispute about the aetiology of the condition, there is also dispute as to whether the classical microscopic appearance of the cochlea is caused by increased endolymph pressure or if this appearance represents an end stage of the process. The mechanism for tinnitus production is even more obscure. If the pressure within the organ of Corti is raised this may cause mechanical disruption and hence cause depolarization of hair cells. However, it is also possible that the process causes rupture of Reissener's membrane with consequent mixing of endolymph and perilymph. This would result in electrolyte changes that could cause depolarization of hair cells. End stage Ménière's disease is characterized by loss of hair cells, though this is often the stage of the disease when tinnitus becomes most troublesome.

The management of Ménière's disease is equally obscure. Medical treatments include:

- a low salt diet
- betahistine

Table 4.1 Causes of endolymphatic hydrops

Congenital:
    some forms of congenital deafness, such as Pendred's syndrome
    cochlear dysplasias, such as Mondini and Scheibe

Trauma:
    head injuries
    surgery

Infection:
    systemic
        syphilis
        mumps
        measles
    otic
        labyrinthitis

Neoplasia:
    leukaemia
    Letterer-Siwe disease

Immunological:
    autoimmune sudden sensorineural hearing loss
    Cogan's syndrome

Bone disease:
    otosclerosis
    Paget's disease

- diuretics
- vestibular sedatives.

Surgery (conservative procedures) include:

- endolymphatic sac surgery: some surgeons decompress the sac whereas others insert a shunt tube or even excise it in an attempt to stabilize endolymph pressure in the inner ear
- grommet insertion: there is no logical basis for inserting a grommet in the management of Ménière's disease but the procedure is still undertaken; any benefit that does arise may well be attributed to the placebo effect.

Surgery (destructive procedures) include:

- intratympanic gentamicin: this uses the fact that gentamicin is more toxic to the neuroepithelium of the vestibular apparatus than the cochlea to ablate residual vestibular function without damaging the hearing

- vestibular nerve section
- labyrinthectomy.

There are some indications that patients with Ménière's disease have specific tinnitus experiences. Stouffer and Tyler (1990) noted that patients with Ménière's disease had significantly higher ratings of tinnitus severity and annoyance than patients with other aetiologies. Douek and Reid (1968) found that patients with tinnitus as a symptom of Ménière's disease consistently matched their tinnitus to a low frequency tone (usually in the range 125–250 Hz) unlike the majority of tinnitus patients who match tinnitus to a pitch above 3000 Hz (Tyler, 2000). Erlandsson et al. (1996) noted that those patients with anxiety and depression associated with Ménière's disease found their tinnitus intolerable.

Most research into Ménière's disease has tended to concentrate primarily on the vertiginous symptoms and secondarily on the hearing loss. There is less information about the effects of the various treatments on any tinnitus. Research on the various medical treatments suggested that they improved the dizziness but had little effect on the other symptoms. Endolymphatic sac surgery may help the tinnitus in a few patients. A recent review article looked at the effects of vestibular nerve section on tinnitus in Ménière's disease. Overall, a mean of 16.4% had worse tinnitus post-operatively, 38.5% were unchanged and 37.2% felt their tinnitus improved (Baguley et al., 2002). A note of caution is sounded by Vernon and Johnson (1980), who found that following vertigo control some patients with Ménière's disease focus more upon their tinnitus and hence are more distressed by it.

Vestibular schwannomas

Although these benign tumours were previously known as 'acoustic neuromas' they should more correctly be called vestibular schwannomas as the tumours are not true neuromas and generally arise on one of the vestibular nerves rather than the auditory nerve. Patients generally complain of unilateral hearing loss and tinnitus. Although these benign tumours arise on the vestibular nerve their growth is so gradual that the patient has time to accommodate to the changing vestibular input, and balance symptoms are less common than hearing symptoms. However, these lesions can on occasion mimic other conditions: vestibular schwannomas have been reported with symptoms suggestive of acute vestibular failure, benign paroxysmal positional vertigo or Ménière's disease (Morrison and Sterkers, 1996). Investigation is by magnetic resonance imaging. If magnetic resonance imaging is not possible, computed tomography is a useful alternative though is not quite as sensitive. The incidence of vestibular schwannomas has shown an apparent increase but this is probably a reflection of higher indices of suspicion and the availability of better diagnostic tools such as magnetic resonance imaging scanners (Figure 4.1). A recent study suggested an annual incidence of two per 100 000 population (Moffat et al., 1995). This is probably still an underestimate. The pathogenesis is unknown in the majority of cases. It has been suggested that there is an area of cellular instability on the outer covering of the vestibular nerves which predisposes these particular nerves to develop schwannomas. There is a clear genetic cause in a small sub-group of vestibular schwannoma patients who have neurofibromatosis 2 (NF2).

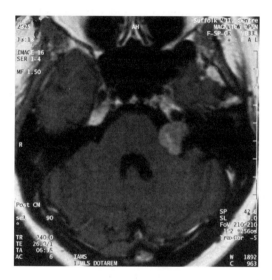

Figure 4.1 A gadolinium-enhanced magnetic resonance imaging scan of a moderate-sized left vestibular schwannoma.

Although from first principles vestibular schwannomas would be expected to cause a retrocochlear or neural deafness, this is not always the case. Purely retrocochlear, purely cochlear or mixed losses can occur. There are various theories as to how vestibular schwannomas cause tinnitus (Baguley et al., 2001).

- Pressure on the auditory nerve causing a physiological breakdown of the insulating properties of the individual nerve fibres with resultant cross-talk between the fibres (ephaptic coupling) (Møller, 1984; Eggermont, 1990; Levine and Kiang, 1995). This theory is discussed in more detail in Chapter 3.
- Pressure on the auditory nerve causing an increase in the desynchronized pseudo-random firing of the auditory nerve (stochastic resonance) (Baguley, 1997; Jastreboff, 1998). This theory is also discussed in more detail in Chapter 3.
- Pressure on the auditory nerve fibres causing destruction of those nerve fibres and hence a block to auditory input. Central tinnitus then supervenes.

- Pressure on the inferior vestibular nerve causing interference with the efferent nerve supply to the cochlea with resultant reduced cochlear 'damping' (Sahley et al., 1997).
- Cochlear tinnitus caused by: pressure on the arterial blood supply causing atrophy of the cochlea; biochemical degradation of the cochlea and the vestibular labyrinth by polypeptides produced by the tumour.

These theories remain unproven. It is probable that the causation of the tinnitus is not the same in every patient with vestibular schwannoma, and more than one pathophysiological process may be at work in any given patient. There are several potential management strategies for patients with vestibular schwannomas:

- do nothing because of age or general health
- watch and wait, offering active treatment only if the lesion grows
- surgery to excise the tumour
- fractionated radiotherapy
- radiosurgery (gamma knife): this is very precise stereotactic radiotherapy that is usually given as a single relatively large dose.

The only one of these treatment options that has good information about tinnitus outcome is the surgical option. Intriguingly, in many cases the tinnitus persists after surgical removal of the tumour (*see* Baguley et al., 2001 for a review) being persistently present in 60% of patients undergoing translabyrinthine removal. Reports indicate that this post-operative tinnitus is severe in a proportion of cases, ranging from 2.5% (Baguley et al., 1992) to 6% (Andersson et al., 1997). As with pre-operative tinnitus, the mechanism of post-operative tinnitus remains unclear: of the hypotheses mentioned above, that of ephaptic coupling could be applied to the post-operative situation as cross-talk has been demonstrated in damaged peripheral nerves (Seltzer and Devor, 1979). Tumour removal necessitates section of the inferior and superior vestibular nerves and so efferent dysfunction will be total because of the ablation of efferent fibres within the inferior vestibular nerve. However, an argument against this being a significant factor in tinnitus persistence is found in studies which indicate that a patient undergoing successful hearing preservation surgery to remove a vestibular schwannoma is less likely to have post-operative tinnitus than one undergoing translabyrinthine surgery (Catalano and Post, 1996). When such hearing preservation surgery is successful, cochlear nerve function is by definition preserved, but the vestibular nerve is sectioned (and thus efferent input ablated) as the tumour is removed.

There is as yet insufficient data on tinnitus and stereotactic radiotherapy. Similarly, there are few data relating to what happens to tinnitus during a 'watch and wait policy', though anecdotally it does seem possible to help this group with tinnitus retraining therapy or psychological treatments.

Pulsatile tinnitus

Pulsatile tinnitus is experienced as a rhythmical noise which may have the same rate as the heart beat. With most forms of tinnitus it is rare to find a single identifiable cause for the problem. With pulsatile tinnitus it is also unusual to find a specific cause but the chances are greater in this form of tinnitus than in the non-pulsatile form. It therefore represents an important sub-group that merits detailed investigation.

Pulsatile tinnitus is sub-divided into subjective (heard only by the patient) and objective (audible to others, either directly, with a stethoscope or with a microphone in the ear canal).

Pulsatile tinnitus is usually caused by a change in blood flow in the vessels near the ear or by a change in awareness of that blood flow. The involved vessels include the large arteries and veins of the neck and base of the skull and smaller vessels within the ear itself.

The blood flow can be altered by a variety of factors.

- Generalized increased blood flow throughout the body, such as occurs in strenuous exercise or severe anaemia. Certain drugs such as angiotensin-converting enzyme inhibitors or calcium channel blockers, used in the treatment of hypertension, heart failure and angina, can cause a hyperdynamic circulation with consequent pulsatile tinnitus.
- Localized increased flow. This can occur when a blood vessel becomes blocked and other neighbouring blood vessels have to carry extra blood or when there are abnormal vessels, such as occurs with arterio-venous malformations. If a blood vessel is stenosed but not completely blocked, blood has to speed up to pass through the stenosed segment. This is seen in atherosclerotic disease of the carotid arteries, and in fibromuscular dysplasia. An atherosclerotic stenosis of the internal carotid artery is shown in Figure 4.2. Vascular tumours such as glomus tumours can increase local blood flow. Metabolically active bone in otosclerosis has a much larger blood supply than normal bone, generating increased local blood flow.
- Turbulent blood flow. If the inside of a blood vessel becomes irregular due to atherosclerosis the blood flow will become turbulent rather than smooth.
- Awareness can be increased by several factors: conductive hearing losses such as perforated eardrums or glue ear tend to make patients more aware of sounds inside their body (somatosounds) because they no longer have the masking effect of external sound; heightened sensitivity in the auditory pathways can alert the brain to normal noise in blood vessels in much the same way that the awareness of non-pulsatile tinnitus is generated.

In addition to the above mechanisms, pulsatile tinnitus is sometimes associated with an enigmatic condition called benign intracranial hypertension or 'pseudo-tumour cerebri'. This unusual syndrome is characterized by

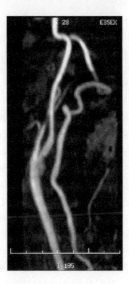

Figure 4.2 MRA of the carotid arteries showing stenosis of the internal carotid artery just above the bifurcation of the common carotid artery.

headaches, dizziness, pulsatile tinnitus, hearing loss and aural fullness: these symptoms may be excerbated on lying down. It is more common in women than men and is frequently associated with obesity. Focal neurological signs are rare apart from occasional VIth or VIIth cranial nerve palsies. Papilloedema is common but not invariable. Magnetic resonance imaging scans may show the typical features of raised intracranial pressure with small cerebral ventricles and effacement of the cortical sulci but this also is not invariable. If the condition is clinically suspected and other causes such as intracranial space-occupying lesions have been excluded diagnosis is confirmed by performing a lumbar puncture and finding raised cerebrospinal fluid pressure with an opening pressure of 200 mm H_2O or more (Sismanis, 1987). Although the condition is idiopathic it is sometimes seen with other disease processes, including hyperthyroidism, anaemia, Cushing's disease and several vitamin deficiencies (Fishman, 1980). It is also seen in patients taking a variety of drugs including some antibiotics, female sex hormones, some non-steroidal anti-inflammatory drugs and steroids (Fishman, 1980; Sismanis, 1987). Treatment is by addressing any associated disease process or medication, encouraging weight loss and judicious use of diuretics (Sismanis and Smoker, 1994).

The investigation of patients with pulsatile tinnitus depends on the clinical history and findings (Weissman and Hirsch, 2000) but generally relies on one or more of the following modalities:

- ultrasound, with Doppler to show the blood flow within vessels
- computed tomography scanning
- magnetic resonance imaging

- magnetic resonance angiography
- angiography, although this is still the most accurate method of investigating the cranial vasculature it is an invasive process with an associated morbidity and mortality, and it is probably no longer justifiable to perform this as a first-line investigation.

An algorithm for the investigation of pulsatile tinnitus is shown in Figure 4.3. The treatment of pulsatile tinnitus clearly depends on the aetiology. High blood pressure can be treated with medication; drug-induced pulsatile tinnitus can be reduced by altering the offending medication, and stenotic segments of carotid artery can be repaired surgically. Vascular tumours, such as glomus tumours (Figure 4.4) or meningiomas, can be excised or if inoperable can be partially controlled with radiotherapy. Otitis media with effusion can be treated with grommets; perforations can be closed with tympanoplasty grafts. For patients with pulsatile tinnitus who have no demonstrable abnormality, methods such as tinnitus retraining therapy or psychological treatments can be used.

Myoclonus

Middle ear myoclonus

The muscles attached to the ossicles can cause an unusual form of tinnitus in which there is rhythmical contraction of the stapedius or tensor tympani muscles giving rise to a fluttering sensation. Where one is confident that the tensor tympani alone is involved the term 'tensor tympani syndrome' may be utilized (Klockhoff, 1981). Diagnosis is from the history and careful examination of the eardrum under magnification. The aetiology is unknown, but a co-incidence with symptoms of stress and anxiety have been noted. Treatments that have been tried include surgical division of the muscle tendons or use of botulinum toxin to paralyse the muscles (Badia et al., 1994). Given the association with sympathetic autonomic nervous system arousal, relaxation therapy or biofeedback (see Chapter 11) may be applied.

Palatal myoclonus

The muscles of the soft palate, some of which are also attached to the Eustachian tube, can also produce tinnitus by rhythmical contraction. Again the aetiology is obscure but in some cases seems to be part of a more widespread neurological condition. The sound may be audible to others. The movement of the palate may be visible. Use of a flexible fibreoptic endoscope is useful here, introduced through the nose to examine the palate from above. This allows the examination to be performed with the patient's mouth shut – the palatal movement is sometimes abolished by mouth opening. Reassurance, anti-epileptic medication and botulinum toxin

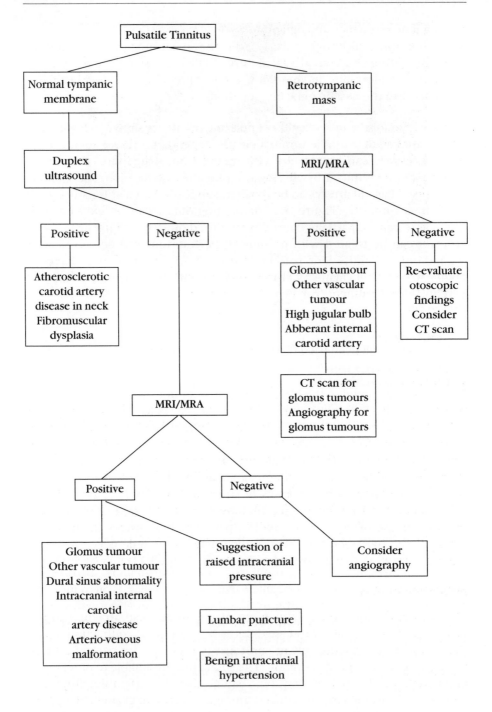

Figure 4.3 An algorithm for the investigation of pulsatile tinnitus. CT = computed tomography; MRA = magnetic resonance angiography; MRI = magnetic resonance imaging.

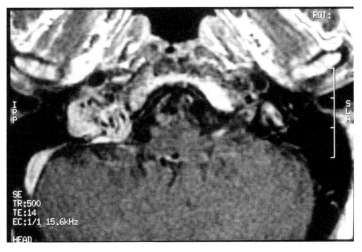

Figure 4.4 Magnetic resonance imaging scan of a right-sided Fisch Type D glomus tumour. The scan shows black flow voids that give the lesion its characteristic 'salt and pepper' appearance.

injections have all been tried (Saeed and Brookes, 1993).

Patulous Eustachian tube

The Eustachian tube spends most of its time closed, opening to equalize the pressure in the middle ear with that in the environment only during swallowing or yawning. There is a rare condition in which the Eustachian tube is abnormally open. During breathing a venturi effect sucks the eardrum medially, giving the patient a sensation of aural fullness, autophony and a flapping sensation. The condition often starts after sudden weight loss and there is often an associated sensorineural hearing loss. Diagnosis is chiefly from the history but careful examination of the tympanic membrane while the patient breathes in and out can show the movement. Measurement of middle ear impedance during respiration can also demonstrate the movement. Treatment is not straightforward. Unfortunately, many of the symptoms are similar to those of glue ear and the condition is often mistaken for Eustachian tube dysfunction or, in other words, an abnormally *closed* Eustachian tube. Having made the wrong diagnosis, the error is compounded by inserting a grommet that tends to exacerbate the problem. Once the condition has been correctly diagnosed there are several therapeutic options: various materials such as Teflon have been injected around the opening of the tube in the nasopharynx to try to close it sufficiently to stop the symptom but not so much that the tube becomes completely blocked (Pulec, 1967). Robinson and Hazell (1989) reported use of controlled diathermy of the medial end of the tube to achieve the same result.

Spontaneous otoacoustic emissions

Most spontaneous otoacoustic emissions are inaudible except with the use of sophisticated instruments. The role of such small amplitude spontaneous otoacoustic emissions in the genesis of tinnitus is dicussed in Chapter 3. However, a very small number of spontaneous otoacoustic emissions are loud enough to be clearly heard by others (Schloth and Zwicker, 1983; Fritsch et al., 2001). Occurring chiefly in children, these large spontaneous otoacoustic emissions have been reported as a cause of objective tinnitus. However, in many cases, although onlookers may be aware of the sound, the patient is often unaware of it. It is therefore a moot point as to whether this should be regarded as tinnitus. Hearing is usually unaffected. Management is generally a thorough explanation of cochlear and particularly outer hair cell function. The patient and relatives should be strongly reassured that there is no serious underlying pathology and that these audible spontaneous otoacoustic emissions tend to fade with time. Low-dose aspirin has been shown to be effective in abolishing the sound in some cases (Fritsch et al., 2001). However, aspirin should not be given to patients under the age of 16 years as there is a risk of precipitating Reye's syndrome.

Temporomandibular disorder and tinnitus

Temporomandibular disorder, also known as 'temporomandibular pain-dysfunction disorder' or 'craniofacial disorder' is defined as symptoms arising from the temporomandibular joints, muscles of mastication and associated structures (McNeill, 1993). Like tinnitus, temporomandibular disorder is common: prevalence is reported as up to 20% of the population. Symptoms and signs of temporomandibular disorder include pain and tenderness around the temporomandibular joints and muscles of mastication; headaches, clicking and crepitus of the temporomandibular joints, locking of the temporomandibular joints, abnormal bite and altered sensation in the face. In addition, temporomandibular disorder can be associated with tinnitus, vertigo, otalgia and altered hearing perception (Chan and Reade, 1994). With two such common conditions as temporomandibular disorder and tinnitus, it is inevitable that some patients should have both conditions and some reports have suggested that such simultaneous occurrence of tinnitus and temporomandibular disorder is just coincidence (Brookes et al., 1980). However, other workers have suggested that there is evidence of a higher than expected prevalence of tinnitus in temporomandibular disorder patients and vice versa (Rubenstein et al., 1990; Rubinstein, 1993). This association of aural symptoms with dysfunction of the temporomandibular joints was first described by Costen in 1934, and the combination of temporomandibular disorder and tinnitus is still sometimes referred to as Costen's syndrome. The pathophysiological processes that link temporomandibular disorder to tinnitus remain obscure but several theories have been proposed. These include common embryological origin of temporomandibular joints and aural structures, shared sensory nerve supply, muscles of mastication acting on the Eustachian tube and ligaments that are common to both the malleus and the temporomandibular joints (Ash and Pinto, 1991; Chen and Reade, 1994). Additionally, the hypothesis of Levine (1999) regarding the influence of somatic systems upon auditory gain and tinnitus may be implicated.

Stomatognatic (dental and jaw) treatment has been studied with relevance to tinnitus, mostly by dentists with a particular interest in tinnitus (Rubinstein and Carlsson, 1987). Non-surgical treatment of tempero-mandibular disorder includes analgesics and anti-inflammatory drugs, anxiolytics and antidepressants. Bite-raising orthodontic splints are helpful in preventing excessive muscle contraction and bruxism. Adoption of a soft diet also helps to reduce strain on the temporomandibular joints. Relaxation therapy and stress management techniques have been used to good effect in temporomandibular disorder (Turk et al., 1996). Surgery is appropriate only when conservative measures have failed. The two commonly used surgical techniques are temporomandibular joint arthroscopy (Steigerwald et al., 1996) and arthrotomy. Both techniques aim to repair damaged structures within the temporomandibular joints. Arthroscopy employs a small endoscope to access the joint, whereas arthrotomy formally opens the joint. Arthrotomy allows more extensive work to be undertaken but is a more invasive procedure and the post-operative recovery period is longer. There have been several studies that have shown that treatment of temporomandibular disorder improves associated tinnitus (Gelb and Bernstein, 1983; Erlandsson et al., 1991). Wright and Bifano (1997) reviewed the relevant literature and concluded that between 46% and 96% of patients with temporomandibular disorder and tinnitus had reduction of the tinnitus when the temporomandibular disorder was treated with splints, although there were methodological flaws in most of the studies. The mechanism by which treating temporomandibular disorder results in reduction of any associated tinnitus remains obscure, though Campbell (1993) suggested that large doses of non-steroidal anti-inflammatory drugs are often used to alleviate the symptoms of temporomandibular disorder and these might in fact exacerbate tinnitus. Successful treatment of the underlying condition would allow reduction or cessation of non-steroidal anti-inflammatory drug intake with consequent relief of tinnitus.

Unilateral sudden sensorineural hearing loss

A sudden sensorineural hearing loss is considered to be an otological emergency (Arts, 1998; Hughes, 1998) and to necessitate urgent treatment. Little attention has been paid, however, to the consequence to the patient of a sudden sensorineural hearing loss in terms of tinnitus handicap.

The perceived hearing handicap of patients with unilateral hearing loss has been considered (Newman et al., 1997). A series of 43 patients with unilaterally normal hearing completed the Hearing Handicap Inventory for Adults (Newman et al., 1990). It was noted that almost three-quarters (73%) reported mild or greater hearing handicap, which was indicative of 'communication and psychosocial problems', despite the normal contralateral ear. The patients were recruited from otolaryngology outpatients, but it was not recorded for how long they had experienced the unilateral hearing loss, nor if the loss had been gradual or sudden. It might be expected that the sudden and possibly traumatic onset of a unilateral hearing loss might involve more handicap than a loss of insidious onset.

A recent study (Chiossoine-Kerdel et al., 2000) investigated the tinnitus handicap associated with sudden sensorineural hearing loss in a group of patients who were treated in a teaching hospital department of otolaryngology using the Hearing Handicap Inventory for Adults and the Tinnitus Handicap Inventory (Newman et al., 1996) as outcome measures. Tinnitus was reported by 14 of the 21 patients who responded to the postal questionnaires from a total of 38 patients identified as having undergone a sudden sensorineural hearing loss in the years 1988-1997. The median total THI score for those with tinnitus was 20 (interquartile range 52), and in four patients of the 14 with tinnitus (28.6 %) the tinnitus handicap was moderate or severe. The onset of tinnitus was coincident with sudden sensorineural hearing loss in eight patients (57% of the 14 with tinnitus) and occurred within 48 hours in the remaining six (43%). In 18 patients (86% of the 21 patients) a significant hearing handicap was demonstrated by the Hearing Handicap Inventory for Adults score.

The management of sudden sensorineural hearing loss remains controversial. The condition should be thoroughly investigated in an attempt to identify specific treatable pathology (Table 4.2). Many different treatment regimes have been tried but there is no convincing evidence that any are effective when the aetiology of the sudden sensorineural hearing loss is unknown. The medical treatment protocol for idiopathic sudden sensorineural hearing loss used in Addenbrookes Hospital, Cambridge, UK is shown in Table 4.3. Probably of much more benefit is the early support and rehabilitation of both the hearing loss and tinnitus, using hearing therapy and amplification as appropriate.

Summary

There are several well-defined diseases that have tinnitus as part of the symptom complex. Also there are various drugs that are known to induce tinnitus. The mechanisms by which tinnitus is generated in these situations have been well investigated and in most cases are much better understood than in the more commonly encountered non-syndromic tinnitus. From first principles it would be expected that a good understanding of the

Table 4.2 Investigations for sudden sensorineural hearing loss*

Haematology
   full blood count
   erythrocyte sedimentation rate
   clotting screen

Biochemistry
   blood sugar
   urea and electrolytes
   cholesterol/triglycerides
   thyroid function test
   liver function tests

Clinical immunology
   auto-antibodies
   immunoglobulins (IgG, IgM, IgA)
   rheumatoid factors (latex agglutination, Rose Waaler)
   cryoglobulins
   circulating immunocomplexes
   complement profile (C1150, C3, C4, Clq)

Microbiology/serology
   viral antibodies, including Epstein–Barr virus and cytomegalovirus
   syphilis serology
   toxoplasma serology
   Rickettsia serology

Audiology
   daily pure tone audiometry (AC/BC)
   electronystagmography and calorics
   brainstem evoked response audiometry

Radiology
   magnetic resonance imaging scan of internal auditory canals and brain

*Not all these investigations are appropriate to every patient with sudden sensorineural hearing loss and the tests should be tailored to meet the individual patient's requirements.

Table 4.3 Treatment protocol used in the management of sudden sensorineural hearing loss at Addenbrooke's Hospital, Cambridge, UK

Admission to the otolaryngology ward for bedrest

Prednisolone 60 mg daily in four divided doses, for 10 days, slowly reducing over a two-week period

Naftidrofuryl oxalate (Praxilene) 100 mg tds for two weeks

Dextran 40, given as intravenous infusion, 2000 ml per day, reduced to 1500 ml per day if renal or cardiac impairment are present, for 48 hours

If herpes virus aetiology suspected, intravenous acyclovir 5–10 mg /kg tds for up to seven days

Outpatient follow-up at four weeks with full audiometry

pathophysiology should lead to enhanced treatment options and a greater chance of controlling or curing the symptom. However, in practice, the results of treating such conditions are often rather disappointing with regard to tinnitus control. This supports the neurophysiological and psychological models of tinnitus, both of which suggest that although peripheral otological disease may trigger tinnitus, central auditory processes and related systems of reaction and emotion are more important in the distress and long-term effects of the symptom.

Chapter 5
Psychological and neurophysiological models of tinnitus

As a mechanistic view of tinnitus has consistently failed to provide a clinical solution to the problem, in the last quarter of the twentieth century attention was diverted away from specific lesions within the auditory system and redirected towards the role of the central nervous system in tinnitus distress. This thinking gave rise to psychological and neurophysiological models of tinnitus that have supplied the rationale for most currently utilized therapeutic interventions.

Psychological habituation model

In 1984 Richard Hallam and colleagues (including Ronald Hinchcliffe, an eminent neuro-otologist) presented a compelling psychological model of tinnitus. These workers observed that most cases of tinnitus are associated with 'some neurophysiological disturbance in the auditory system at any point between periphery and cortex' (Hallam et al., 1984: 33). However, they also noted that some cases of tinnitus occur without aural pathology, citing the findings of Heller and Bergman (1953), in which people who stated that they had no hearing impairment and no previous tinnitus reported hearing tinnitus-like noises when placed in a soundproof environment. Hallam et al. (1984) went on to suggest that psychological processes were involved in tinnitus and, as well as psychological factors affecting tinnitus, the converse could also happen. This suggestion of both psychosomatic and somatopsychic interactions echoed the findings of previous work by Tyler and Baker (1983), and indeed work by Fowler (1948), in which clear psychosomatic links were proposed. Hallam et al. (1984) suggested that efficient central neural processing requires selective inhibition of sensory input, and that this process may be impaired when the attentional system is required to process excessive levels of input, in particular during states of high central nervous system and autonomic nervous system arousal. They further suggested that tinnitus does not receive continuous conscious attention and can be modified by factors such as masking, distraction and

55

changes in arousal, including circadian rhythm. Hallam (1987) further elaborated on the role of self-attentiveness in the development of tinnitus distress.

Hallam et al. (1984) observed that the majority of people who experience tinnitus do not complain about the symptom and suggested that the normal situation is for people to habituate to their tinnitus. Work by Tyler and Baker (1983) supported this hypothesis by showing that the range and intensity of tinnitus-related problems decreased with time, and that there was also no correlation between perceived loudness of the tinnitus and the degree of distress. Habituation has been defined as 'a decrease in response to a benign stimulus when that stimulus is presented repeatedly' (Kandel et al., 2000), and is described in work by Pavlov and by Sherrington (*see* Kandel et al., 2000 for a review). Using Horvath's (1980) rules of habituation, Hallam and colleagues (1984) postulated that tinnitus should rapidly lose its novelty and habituation should occur, but that in certain situations this process could be expected not to occur. Such situations include high levels of autonomic nervous system arousal, sudden onset of tinnitus, particularly intense aversive or unpredictable tinnitus or if the tinnitus develops emotional significance through a learning process (Groves and Thompson, 1970). Habituation could also be affected if the neural pathways involved in habituation were damaged. Conversely, tinnitus awareness could be attributed to dishabituation of a previously tolerated signal because of psychological change.

In this model it was further proposed that an orienting response to tinnitus could interrupt normal behaviour, thereby increasing arousal and consequently reducing habituation. This would produce a pathophysiological positive feedback loop, resulting in persistence of the symptom. This proposal is supported by the observation that tinnitus distress tends to increase in quiet environments where the signal (tinnitus) to noise (background sound) ratio is greater. Extending this theory, Hallam et al. (1984) suggested that anything that alters the signal to noise ratio may affect tinnitus perception and that distress will increase as awareness of the tinnitus interferes with normal central neural activity.

This model can be used to develop treatment strategies. First, reducing levels of autonomic system arousal would be expected to be beneficial. This is generally achieved by relaxation therapy. Second, changing the emotional meaning of tinnitus should reduce the distress. This can be achieved by formal cognitive therapy, but also by vouchsafing information about the mechanisms of tinnitus and associated distress. Formal psychological treatments are discussed in more depth in Chapter 13.

Neurophysiological model

Having reviewed potential physiological mechanisms of tinnitus, Jastreboff (1990) presented a neurophysiological model of tinnitus. This was based on the tenet that, in addition to the classical auditory system pathways, other central neural pathways are involved in the emergence and maintenance of tinnitus. In particular, the limbic system, sympathetic autonomic nervous system and reticular formation are pivotal to the hypothesis. Jastreboff proposed that signal recognition and classification circuits are involved in persistent tinnitus, as neural networks that become tuned to the tinnitus signal, even when that signal is of low intensity or intermittent. Peripheral processes might indeed be involved in the generation of tinnitus-related activity, but bearing in mind the findings of Heller and Bergman (1953), it was not necessary for an auditory system dysfunction to be present for tinnitus to be perceived. This Jastreboff 'neurophysiological model', was published in diagrammatic form in 1996 and in slightly more detailed form in 1999 (Figure 5.1).

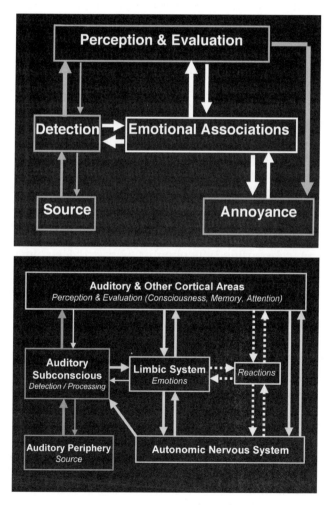

Figure 5.1 Diagrammatic representation of the Jastreboff neurophysiological model. Arrows denote interrelations between different functional areas of the auditory system.

It was noted that after a short period of awareness of tinnitus-related activity, a process of habituation may occur so that the activity is no longer consciously perceived. However, in cases where there is some 'negative emotional reinforcement', described as fear, anxiety or tension, then limbic system and sympathetic autonomic activation cause the activity to be enhanced and perception persists. The distinction between the perception and the behavioural and emotional reaction to tinnitus was explicit, as was the potential for a feedback loop between these processes.

The Jastreboff neurophysiological model suggests that, in tinnitus, the links between these elements of the central nervous system are governed by classical conditioning or associative learning (Schwartz, 1989). Although not described in detail by Jastreboff, these processes are based on Aristotle's third principle of contiguity. This states that if two or more experiences occur together frequently enough then eventually one occurring on its own will evoke memory of the other(s). The most famous examples of this are Pavlov's experiments (1927), in which a neutral stimulus (a bell ringing) was presented to dogs at the same time as they were given another stimulus (food) which naturally produced salivation. After a while the dogs salivated when the bell was rung even if no food was present. The presentation of food was the natural or unconditioned stimulus; the bell ringing was the neutral stimulus or conditioned stimulus; the salivation without the presence of food was the conditioned reflex. Jastreboff (1999) suggested that tinnitus becomes a problem when it becomes associated with negative experiences, though he did not clearly elaborate upon what comprises the unconditioned stimulus, the conditioned stimulus and the conditioned response in that process. Although the negative experience may be a change within the auditory system, it may also be an unrelated stressful event such as bereavement, relationship difficulties or work problems. Indeed, Jastreboff (1999) suggested that in the majority of cases of tinnitus the emergence is not related to auditory system change. Negative information or beliefs about tinnitus can supply negative reinforcement, which, via the limbic system, stimulates the sympathetic arm of the autonomic nervous system releasing catecholamines and producing a fight or flight response. Because this autonomic response is unpleasant, it in turn acts as further negative reinforcement.

There are several points within the auditory, reactive and emotional systems where feedback can occur. One of the main feedback pathways occurs in the lower part of the model (Figure 5.1) between the auditory subconscious, the limbic system and the autonomic nervous system. This lower loop operates at a pre-conscious level. An upper feedback loop also involves the limbic system and the autonomic nervous system but in addition incorporates higher cortical centres and hence operates at a conscious level. Jastreboff (1999) suggested that the lower loop is dominant in most people who have severe tinnitus. The neurophysiological model hypothesis also suggests that once the central feedback loops have become established the auditory periphery becomes relatively unimportant. There is evidence to support this as section of the auditory nerve fails to control severe established tinnitus in up to 50% of cases (*see* Chapter 11).

Jastreboff et al. (1996) used this neurophysiological model to develop a treatment strategy called tinnitus retraining therapy (*see* Chapter 12), but has subsequently been careful of late to state that tinnitus retraining therapy is not the only treatment that is congruent with the neurophysiological model. The model itself has been criticized for being oversimplistic (Andersson, 2002a), but this is perhaps to miss the point: in that simplicity lies the ease of communication to patients and indeed to non-specialist clinicians.

Evidence for both models

Unfortunately, surprisingly little research has followed the important theoretical contributions of Hallam et al. (1984). In many respects this is also the case with the Jastreboff neurophysiological model if one looks for experimental evidence relating to human experiences. The neurophysiological model does have some support from animal studies (Jastreboff and Sasaki, 1994).

One possible reason for confusion with regard to the habituation model is that Hallam and colleagues concentrated on cognitive habituation processes that described habituation of reaction, whereas most research studies have considered psychophysiological measures of habituation, such as skin conductance and event-related potentials (*see* Chapter 7). Carlsson and Erlandsson (1991), for example, studied 14 patients of whom seven were complainers and seven non-complainers, measuring skin conductance and heart rate changes in response to a series of tinnitus-like sounds. No differences in habituation were observed, but in fact some signs of opposite mechanisms (e.g. sensitization) were found in the complainer group. Complainers compared with non-complainers increased their heart rate. For many reasons this small-scale study cannot be regarded as a fair test of the habituation model. Walpurger et al. (2003) (*see* Chapter 7) tested Hallam's habituation model and found some support for a lack of habituation to tone pips by use of auditory evoked potentials. Other previous experiments on evoked potentials have also been interpreted as showing evidence of habituation failure (Attias et al., 1993a). When it comes to psychological habituation (e.g. caring less about it) the evidence is mixed, as older adults with longstanding tinnitus may have more instead of less severe annoyance (*see* Chapter 2).

The assertions made in the neurophysiological model are also not as well supported as sometimes claimed. For example, it is not clear that tinnitus can be likened to a tone, to which the patient is classically conditioned. Further, the role of the limbic system in tinnitus distress might seem hard to contest, but indeed imaging research has not been fully consistent with this theory (Chapter 7). Indeed, from a learning psychology point of view, there is much left to explain within the neurophysiological model, such as the temporal properties and actual instances when aversive reactions have become conditioned (McKenna, 2004).

Given that tinnitus is not viewed as an unconditioned stimulus for unconditioned aversive reactions (which it might very well be: for example, as a sign of becoming deaf), there is a missing link to explain; namely, how a tone without meaning (i.e. tinnitus) becomes paired with an unconditioned aversive stimulus. Here, the Jastreboff model takes a tautological approach and does not explain *why* tinnitus becomes bothersome. Indeed, it might not be classical conditioning that takes place but rather 'evaluative conditioning' (DeHouwer et al., 2001). Evaluative conditioning refers to changes in the liking of a stimulus because the stimulus has been paired with other, positive or negative, stimuli. In evaluative conditioning studies, a neutral stimulus is paired with an affective stimulus and changes in the valence of the neutral stimulus are measured. Interestingly, unlike most forms of Pavlovian conditioning, evaluative conditioning is highly resistant to extinction.

Further elaborations on a psychological model

The models of Hallam and Jastreboff could be completed by basic research into cognitive processing of sounds and of the link between cognition and emotion. Among these neglected areas are selective processing and attention, the effects of tinnitus on memory and information processing, and the emotional processing of tinnitus-related thoughts and experiences (Andersson, 2002a). Research of this kind could illuminate the concept of habituation of reaction (Jastreboff, 2000), as this might be more readily highlighted by cognitive tests (e.g. selective processing of the tinnitus sound) than by self-report measures.

It is possible that working memory is affected by tinnitus (Andersson et al., 2002a; Anderson et al., 2002b). Working memory is the memory system that holds perceptual input while interpretation of it is worked out (Baddeley, 1986). In this context it has been important to investigate the role of background sounds in relation to tinnitus. It is well known that tinnitus often can be covered (masked) by environmental sounds, and that it can in some circumstances be totally masked. However, consideration of masking is complicated by the fact that tinnitus does not 'behave' as an acoustic sound and that it might resurface if one attempts to mask it (Penner et al., 1981). Andersson (2002a) proposed that the 'changing-state' character of the tinnitus signal may increase tinnitus distress. This had been suggested already in the habituation model by Hallam. In brief, experimental literature on the changing-state effect has found that not only speech but also tones that vary in pitch and segmentation disrupt cognitive performance. Although irrelevant sounds can be habituated to, even a brief hiatus has the capacity to restore the disruption (Banbury et al., 2001). Habituation is not likely to occur if the disturbing sound varies in complexity. Even if tinnitus were a stable neural signal (which neuroscience research implies is not the case), it might be a stimulus of changing-state character because of the influence of environmental sounds masking the tinnitus in an unpredictable manner. In a recent review Banbury et al. (2001) outlined the conditions during which cognition is disrupted by irrelevant sounds. They pointed out that both the properties of the sound and of the cognitive task are crucial. Interestingly, loudness of the disrupting sound is not important (as in tinnitus), and neither is the meaning of the sound (e.g. speech disrupts cognition even when in another language). However, there is one caveat: if the degree of change in the auditory stimulus becomes very marked, the degree of disruption can also diminish. This would account for the clinical observation that tinnitus with large variations in sound quality and presence does not appear to be more annoying than tinnitus that is experienced as stable. The brain-imaging literature on tinnitus suggests that tinnitus in many ways is processed as a complex auditory stimulus, involving secondary associative auditory cortex, and areas related to attention (*see* Chapter 7).

The cognitive disruption might serve as a starting point for later conditioned emotional reactions to tinnitus. It is thought that tinnitus has an interfering effect on cognitive function, and that this effect is noted by the person who starts to attend to the tinnitus. Focus on tinnitus leads to less attention to other conflicting sounds (or camouflaging sounds), which might then be perceived as an increase in loudness (or contrast). Fundamental to all such hypotheses is the possibility of emotional responses to tinnitus. This might occur at all points, including when tinnitus first appears, when it is found to disrupt cognitive function and when fluctuations are experienced.

Several authors have proposed that attentional factors may play a crucial role in moderating the adverse effects of tinnitus. For example, Jastreboff (1990: 243), in his seminal paper, wrote 'The psychological components related to the evaluation of tinnitus and the type of emotion it evokes are of particular importance, and the procedures which affect this evaluation are likely to be effective in tinnitus alleviation'. Jacobson et al. (1996) found that tinnitus patients showed evidence of early selective auditory attention by means of an experimental paradigm in which participants were asked to attend and respond to an occasional target stimulus presented in one ear while ignoring information (including the target stimulus) presented in the opposite ear. The role of cognitive processes in tinnitus is yet to be further explored. However, while the changing-state hypothesis looks promising, it needs to be tested in more detail, and the similarities between tinnitus and changing-state stimuli used in the experimental studies by Jones and co-workers (e.g. Jones and Macken, 1993) need further investigation. It is, however, plausible that tinnitus disrupts concentration and that this effect is dependent on the attention given to tinnitus. The changing-state hypothesis could be one of several possible missing links in the attempt to explain why a sound without meaning, like tinnitus, evokes such strong conditioned emotional responses in some people but not in others.

Summary

Although there are many similarities between the psychological and neurophysiological models of tinnitus there are also some important areas of divergence. Both models relegate the cochlea to a minor role in tinnitus distress and give much greater importance to the role of the brain and autonomic nervous system. Both regard emotional processing as the major factor in generating tinnitus distress, and both see habituation as the means of reducing that distress. However, the neurophysiological model regards the subconscious processing of auditory information as being more important than conscious evaluation of the symptom in most patients, whereas the psychological habituation model stresses the importance of conscious beliefs. The differing treatment strategies that these models have provided are discussed in Chapters 12 and 13.

Chapter 6
How tinnitus is perceived and measured

There is a long history of attempts to measure tinnitus (Henry and Meikle, 2000; Tyler, 2000). Perhaps the most influential contribution was by Edmund Prince Fowler in the 1940s (Fowler, 1942), who undertook systematic investigations, but earlier attempts were published by Josephson, (1931) and Wegel (1931). In these two early studies a serious attempt to measure tinnitus was made by means of comparisons with pure tones, a strategy that was later to be used in many studies. However, it was Fowler's work that developed many of the principles that researchers and clinicians still adhere to today. For example, it was Fowler who noted the discrepancy between the reported loudness of tinnitus and the actual loudness measured in sensation level (SL). It was also Fowler (1942, 1944) who discovered that most patients matched their tinnitus loudness to 5 dB SL or 10 dB SL, only a few decibels above their hearing thresholds. This chapter examines the sound quality of tinnitus, how localization can been assessed, the pitch of the tinnitus sound, masking level and, lastly, the effects of masking tinnitus. It is not easy to measure tinnitus and there are many reasons why no standard set of tests has been reached for the psychoacoustical description of tinnitus. Tyler (2000) mentioned three sources of difficulty:

- test–retest variability
- the normal fluctuation of the tinnitus in many patients
- changes in the tinnitus produced by the measurement stimulus in some patients.

In addition, some patients do not have one, but several tinnitus sounds, and these sounds may have different temporal and loudness characteristics.

Sound quality

In order to know how tinnitus is perceived it is important to ask the patient, since no objective way to measure this aspect of tinnitus exists. Some tinnitus patients have a tinnitus that is difficult to describe in words, but it is important to try to understand patients' tinnitus experiences by careful history-taking. The audiometer can be used to try to match patients' tinnitus. Unfortunately, this is not an easy task, and it almost always fails because the sound produced by the audiometer rarely sounds the same as the tinnitus: the tinnitus sound is often too complicated to be replicated by an audiometer. Mitchell et al. (1984) and Penner (1993) studied whether the tinnitus sound could be simulated using a synthesizer, but even this sophisticated technology failed to solve the problem. However, interestingly, Penner (1996) found that there was no real difference between how tinnitus patients and people without tinnitus rated a set of 'tinnitus sounds' in terms of annoyance. These tinnitus sounds had been derived from computer simulation. One conclusion from the study was that tinnitus sounds are perceived as annoying by most people. In one study, reported by Wahlström and Axelsson (1995), 50 normal hearing subjects from an audiology department were asked to describe a set of sounds (pure tones at 250 Hz, 4 KHz and 8 kHz) that were presented via an audiometer at a comfortable sound level for five seconds. The same stimulus material was presented to 50 tinnitus patients. Results showed that tinnitus patients perceived the tones as less clear compared with the normal hearing subjects.

Despite the difficulties in generating tinnitus sounds that exactly match the sensation of tinnitus, there are several reports of how the sounds are described from patients' own words. Stouffer and Tyler (1990) studied over 500 tinnitus patients and found that the most common description was ringing (37%); in second place came whirling (11%); in third place, crickets (9%) and fourth hissing (8%). The remaining descriptions included a large range of different sounds. In another large study of 1800 tinnitus patients, Meikle and Taylor-Walsh (1984) found that 30% of their patients described their tinnitus as 'ringing'. This is a common observation both in clinical practice and in research, with the addition that patients often report a combination of sounds that can sound very different and distinct; for example, a buzzing sound in one ear and a tone in the other ear. In some research there is a brief characterization of tinnitus as either tonal, buzzing or a combination of the two. Douek (1981) proposed that tinnitus could be categorized from patients' own descriptions into: low tones; high whistles; humming machines; multiple sounds; and complex sounds.

Tinnitus patients describe their tinnitus in diverse ways. Sometimes they will find a metaphor for the sound. It is useful for clinicians to ask patients if the tinnitus sounds like anything they have heard previously. Some examples, written by patients from the tinnitus clinic in Uppsala are given in Table 6.1.

Clearly there are many metaphors for tinnitus, but in our experience it is usually the case that tinnitus is not described as something dramatic and interesting. More commonly, tinnitus is likened to mechanical and rather

Table 6.1 Examples of patients' descriptions of tinnitus sounds (Andersson, 2000b)

A soft ringing sound

Like crickets playing (sometimes over 100)

Metallic sound, like from a decoration from a Christmas tree plus some other sounds

Tonal buzzing 'fluorescent tube'

A high tone with a wind in the background

Buzzing. Like someone flushing water

A loud cutting tone surrounded by buzzing in colour

Scream

Rushing

Loud bag-pipe

A high-pitched tone heard all the time

Just as when the television broadcasting ends (buzzing sound)

Buzzing

Like a signal and scream. Persistent most of the time, but sometimes pulsating and jumpy during movement.

Buzzing, like a midge or mosquito

boring sounds. In fact, often patients can only come up with 'ringing sound' as a metaphor for tinnitus. Surprisingly, little systematic research has been devoted to the perception of the tinnitus sound. None of the commonly used tinnitus questionnaires addresses the different aspects of the perceived sound quality of the tinnitus. This is definitely an area that deserves further research as there are useful clinical implications for some patients. In some cases, a more meaningful metaphor for tinnitus (eg diamond drill with a craftsman sitting in a room working) can be used as a way of helping to attain habituation.

Pitch

Pitch matching is undertaken with the objective of trying to generate a sound that matches the tinnitus pitch, which later can be used to estimate tinnitus loudness. This is relevant only in tonal tinnitus. Descriptions dating back to the 1930s have described ways to do this (Josephson, 1931; Wegel, 1931) and further studies have been published subsequently (Tyler and Stouffer, 1978; Henry and Meikle, 2000). Measuring tinnitus pitch is somewhat arduous – for both clinicians and patients. Tinnitus may not be easy to match to a single tone, but according to Tyler and Babin (1993) most patients can at least compare their tinnitus with a tone, or a tone that is part of the whole tinnitus perception.

The use of synthesizers to find a tinnitus tone closer to the tinnitus may not be practical in clinical settings. However, it is possible that computerized assessment of tinnitus will facilitate this (Mitchell et al., 1984; Henry and Meikle, 1999). In addition to clinician-administered tinnitus matching there could be a role for self-generated matching. Summarizing data from several studies, it is common to match tinnitus to a tone at 4000 Hz. The majority of patients describe a pitch that exceeds 3000 Hz. For many patients, tinnitus pitch corresponds to start of the measured hearing loss on their audiogram. This is of theoretical importance given the discordant damage hypothesis put forward by Jastreboff (1990) (*see* Chapter 3).

Obtaining measures of pitch can be done in different ways. Tyler and Conrad-Armes (1983a) compared three ways of assessing pitch and came to the conclusion that it was best to measure pitch from the ear with tinnitus. Others, however, have instead recommended that the contralateral ear should be used for pitch estimates (Henry and Meikle, 2000). In most cases it does not appear to be of major importance if the tinnitus ear or the contralateral ear is used. The process becomes more complicated with bilateral asymmetrical tinnitus. However, there is a consensus that one ear at a time should be tested rather than presenting simultaneous binaural stimuli.

The diagnostic value of tinnitus pitch has been discussed (Douek and Reid, 1968; Tyler and Conrad-Armes, 1983a). For example, in noise-induced hearing loss tinnitus is often high-pitched (Henry and Meikle, 2000), and in the early stages of Ménière's disease tinnitus is reportedly low-pitched (Douek and Reid, 1968; Vernon and Johnson, 1980). However, the use of tinnitus pitch as a diagnostic tool is of questionable value. From a diagnostic point of view it is also important to look at test–retest reliability of pitch estimates, and in this respect the results are far from encouraging (Henry et al., 1999).

Loudness

Many patients want some estimate of the loudness of their tinnitus, which they can use to inform other people of their condition. However, an early observation by Fowler (1942) was the lack of correspondence between patients' views and the obtained loudness estimates. Loudness of tinnitus can be measured in many ways, but most commonly patients are instructed to say when a tone or a broad-band noise reaches the same level as the tinnitus.

One early research finding was that tinnitus, for most patients, matches to sound of low intensities, relative to the threshold of hearing (Fowler, 1942; Reed, 1960; Tyler and Stouffer, 1989). In practical terms, if tinnitus is matched to a tone of 40 dB hearing level (HL), and the patient has a hearing threshold of 35 dB HL for that frequency, the level of tinnitus in terms of sensation level (SL) becomes only 5 dB (40 dB minus 35 dB), which corresponds to a very low-intensity sound. However, describing tinnitus in terms of SL may be inappropriate (Penner and Klafter, 1992), as it is grounded in the concept that tinnitus is just like any other sound or tone. Andersson (2003) reviewed the literature on the differences between expressing tinnitus loudness in HL versus SL, and found that the association with annoyance was stronger for HL. Hence, one alternative would be to describe tinnitus in dBHL. However, this inevitably makes the level of hearing loss part of the definition of loudness, and it is known from epidemiological studies that hearing impairment is significantly associated with both the presence and annoyance of tinnitus. One alternative is to match tinnitus against a tone for which the patient has normal hearing (Goodwin et al., 1980; Penner, 1986), which may result in a more reliable estimate of loudness (Risey et al., 1989).

From a clinical point of view it is often unhelpful to talk about tinnitus in terms of SL, as it implies that the patient is imagining that the tinnitus is loud when it is really not. The title of one of Fowler's papers, 'The "illusion of loudness" of tinnitus', clearly suggests this (Fowler, 1942). Largely because of these practical and theoretical objections, loudness estimates have gone out of fashion in the management of tinnitus.

There are alternative and more complex ways of measuring tinnitus loudness (Hinchcliffe and Chambers, 1983; Matsuhira et al., 1992); for example, by considering the effect of recruitment (non-linear loudness growth). Tyler and Conrad-Armes (1983b) derived a formula for calculating tinnitus loudness correcting for recruitment, which indicates the loudness in 'sones' (a psychoacoustical measure of loudness growth in an individual) (Tyler, 2000). Later research has tended to ignore recruitment as a possible reason for the discrepancy between measured loudness and the experienced annoyance. Even if these alternative ways of obtaining loudness estimates have their advantages, they are rarely used in clinical practice because of time constraints and lack of clinical relevance.

Estimates of the loudness of tinnitus can vary when subjects are retested (Penner, 1983; Burns, 1984), in a similar way to measurements of tinnitus pitch. This variation may reflect poor test–retest reliability of measures or may show that the tinnitus actually changes. Changes in loudness often occur within short time periods, and these variations may be a contributing factor to the tinnitus distress experienced by patients. Tinnitus seems more problematic if patients cannot predict or control the loudness.

It is hard to ignore the fact that one of the most important measures of tinnitus – the perceived intensity – is afflicted with a host of problems. The notion that tinnitus in most cases is a low-intensity sound is problematic as current psychoacoustical measures do not mirror how the brain manages tinnitus (e.g. the cortical representation).

Maskability

Another perspective upon the intrusiveness of tinnitus is to measure the minimal masking level; in other words, the level of sound required for the tinnitus to disappear from awareness. Anecdotally, masking was discovered by

Vernon in the early 1970s (Vernon, 1998), but the knowledge that external sound can mask tinnitus has probably existed for as long as there have been humans with tinnitus (*see* Chapter 1). Overall, the phenomenon of masking has been researched fairly extensively (Henry and Meikle, 2000), with various approaches and interesting findings revealing that tinnitus does not behave as do 'natural' sounds (e.g. tones) in terms of masking characteristics.

The frequency relationship of tinnitus masking effects by means of using tones was investigated in early work by Feldmann (1971), who tested 200 tinnitus patients and investigated how tones with increasing frequencies masked tinnitus, and by doing this generated tinnitus-masking curves. Feldmann found evidence for different types of masking curves. For the first type of masking curve, entitled 'convergent', the threshold curve and the masking curve converge from low to high frequencies (Figure 6.1). Once the tinnitus pitch is reached, the curves converge and follow each other afterwards. From Feldmann's data 34% of patients show this pattern, which was said to be typical of noise-induced hearing loss. The second type, said to be very rare (3%), show the opposite pattern 'divergent', as threshold and masking curves diverge from low to high frequencies. Type three, called the 'congruence' type, was found to be common (32%) and was characterized by the fact that any tone or narrow-band noise, raised above threshold, will mask the tinnitus. The fourth type, 'distance', was seen in 20% of patients and is what many people would expect from annoying tinnitus, that is, threshold curve and masking curve are distant from each other. Type five is the 'resistance' type, when tinnitus is not masked by any kind of sound. In Feldmann's material as many as 11% of patients showed this pattern. These findings and other studies (Tyler and Conrad-Armes, 1984; Tyler, 1987) show that tinnitus is not masked as an ordinary tone, and Henry and Meikle (2000: 149) concluded, 'tinnitus masking appears to be categorically different from the conventional masking of one external tone by another'.

White noise or pink noise can be utilized to mask tinnitus. The question of using broad- versus narrow-band noise as masking for tinnitus has been widely debated. One study by Shailer et al. (1981) found that some patients could benefit from a narrow-band noise, as a lower level of sound was needed to mask the tinnitus. These authors concluded that different patients might prefer different characteristics of the masking sound. Smith et al. (1991) tested this notion and asked 10 experienced tinnitus patients to test and later choose which bandwidth of masking they preferred. They found no convincing evidence that a certain masking sound would be preferred, but interestingly, a majority of patients chose a masking sound that only partially masked their tinnitus. One potential explanation, which corresponds with reports from patients, is that a lower masking sound makes it easier to attend to environmental sound such as conversation, especially if the individual concerned has any degree of hearing loss.

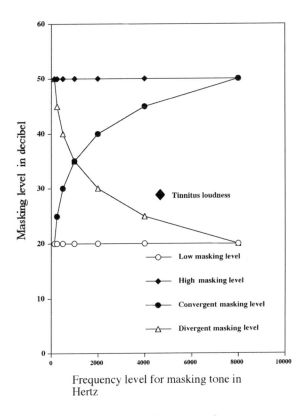

Figure 6.1 Masking curves, based on Feldmann's work.

An important observation by Tyler (1987) is that for many patients the laterality of the masking sound makes no difference. Even if tinnitus is perceived predominantly in the right ear, it can still be masked by a sound in the left ear. This observation suggests that tinnitus is masked at a higher level of the brain, and not at the level of hair cells. This is not a new idea: Minton (1923: 509) suggested that tinnitus masking was probably 'a property of the auditory nerves or even of the acoustic centres of the brain itself'.

Another interesting issue about minimal masking level is that it has been found to respond to treatment (Jastreboff et al., 1994) and to predict long-term outcome (Andersson et al., 2001).

Effects of masking

One remarkable finding in the tinnitus literature is the fact that, for some individuals, tinnitus can disappear for a short period following masking. This phenomenonon is called 'residual inhibition' and was noted by Feldmann

(1971), and has since been much explored by Vernon and co-workers (Vernon and Meikle, 2000). The discovery raised much hope for a cure, but the effect is most often short lived, often just a few minutes (Terry et al., 1983), and the effect is not seen in all patients. In fact, residual inhibition is just one of several possible outcomes after masking. For example, Tyler (1987) found that for some tinnitus patients, tinnitus instead becomes stronger after termination of masking.

One more disturbing finding was explored by Penner et al. (1981), who found that the minimal masking level for tinnitus was raised over test conditions. In a later investigation Penner (1983) further found that increased masking level was associated with increased annoyance. Two explanations for this phenomenon have been considered by Penner. The first is that the masking sound temporarily worsens tinnitus, thus rendering it more noticeable. The second explanation is that auditory adaptation to the masking sound occurs, without any corresponding adaptation to the tinnitus sound (Penner and Bilger, 1988). Masking as a treatment tool is discussed in Chapter 11, although modern methods of tinnitus management suggest that total masking of tinnitus is unhelpful when habituation is the goal.

All the above measurements of tinnitus have demonstrated poor test-retest reliability, but even this is not a constant observation. Some researchers have reported large variability of tinnitus measurements (Burns, 1984), and Penner (1986) even suggested that the reliability of tinnitus measurements was poor because tinnitus seemed to behave as a fluctuating external stimulus. However, in other studies reliability has been more satisfactory (Mitchell et al., 1993).

Summary

The perceived sound quality of tinnitus is very varied but still gives important clinical information for further counselling. Generating data on tinnitus pitch is notoriously difficult, and in practical terms is often restricted to those patients who have tonal tinnitus. When pitch matching is possible, most patients have a pitch that exceeds 3000 Hz. Measurement of tinnitus loudness is also somewhat fraught and there is still considerable debate about the implications of the results of such measurements. In particular, there is poor correlation between the tinnitus SL and annoyance. Masking of tinnitus has been studied in many ways and historically has also been one of the most influential management options. Overall, the measurement of tinnitus is still far from satisfactory and, in particular, the psycholological aspects of tinnitus loudness, pitch and masking have yet to be explored.

Chapter 7
Objective correlates of tinnitus

One of the many challenges in tinnitus research has been the quest for an objective measure of tinnitus perception. There have, of course, been exceptions, such as spontaneous otoacoustic emissions, which are occasionally implicated in tinnitus and can be measured easily. Unfortunately, in these cases, simple measurement of the sound gives no information about the brain's perception of that sound. There have been some recent developments in the search to find objective measures of tinnitus, and there are also some other methods that use indirect measures, such as reaction time and auditory brainstem responses, to draw conclusions about tinnitus.

Reaction time

A few studies have investigated how tinnitus patients respond to sounds in terms of reaction time. Measures of reaction time are not performed without subjects' active participation, but the results can give us some indication as to how the brain processes the tinnitus signal. Goodwin and Johnson (1980b) found that tinnitus patients ($n = 9$) responded faster to tones that matched their tinnitus frequency compared with sounds of a non-tinnitus frequency for which hearing was normal. A significant inter-group difference in reaction times for the tinnitus frequency was also seen when the patients were compared with a control group, with the tinnitus subjects exhibiting more rapid reaction. Nieschalk et al. (1998) partly replicated these findings in a study with 15 tinnitus patients and 15 normal-hearing control subjects. Patients were faster at the tinnitus frequencies and also at the 1000 Hz frequency. In addition, the tinnitus group displayed shorter reaction times at sensation levels near threshold, but no differences for sound stimuli in the suprathreshold region.

It is not easy to explain this effect, and another study found the opposite result (Attias et al., 1996a), with slower reaction times. Nieschalk et al. (1998) considered their findings to be indicative of cochlear dysfunction and went on to suggest that the cochlea could be dysfunctional even when audiometric

71

thresholds are broadly normal (which was the case in their study). However, these authors also pointed out the importance of central processing in tinnitus. Nieschalk et al. (1998) excluded patients with signs of mood disorder from their study. Such mood disorders are common among tinnitus clinic patients (Zöger et al. 2001) and might be expected to influence reaction time. It is therefore difficult to extrapolate the findings of this study to a wider tinnitus group.

Evoked response audiometry

Evoked response audiometry is a set of techniques in which electrical potentials from the brainstem or cerebral cortex are measured by means of electrodes attached to the scalp. The ears are stimulated with sound stimuli (clicks or tone pips) and a summating average of the responses performed by a computer to reflect evoked auditory activity in the brain (Pratt, 2003). In tinnitus research two types of responses to auditory stimuli have been studied. The first type consists of the short latency responses occurring within 10 milliseconds (ms) after the onset of the stimulus. This auditory brainstem response (ABR) consists of five major waveforms, which are thought to reflect electrical activity in auditory pathways at various levels of the brainstem. The second type consists of responses that occur 50–400 ms after stimulus onset and are assumed to reflect cognitive activity, such as auditory attention.

Auditory brainstem responses

There are several studies in which ABR in tinnitus patients has been compared with similar measurements in control subjects who do not have tinnitus. Some studies have given inconclusive results (Barnea et al., 1990; McKee and Stephens, 1992; Attias et al., 1996a), but others have indicated that both early and late ABR waves are affected in tinnitus (Maurizi et al., 1985; Ikner and Hassen, 1990; Rosenhall and Axelsson, 1995). Rosenhall and Axelsson (1995) found delayed latencies for all ABR waves and interpreted these results as indicating brainstem dysfunction rather than impaired hearing. Gerken et al. (2001) studied ABRs and middle latency responses and found that only ABR wave VII was affected in repeated-measures analysis. One problem with this research is that different studies have used very different sample groups, rendering comparison difficult. In addition, there have been no efforts to control for possible psychological factors such as attention.

Cortical evoked potentials

Cortical evoked potentials, in the form of either auditory evoked electrical responses or their magnetic field equivalents (e.g. M100), have been studied in relation to tinnitus, and are of particular interest as they reflect higher-order processing of auditory stimuli. Hoke et al. (1989) found a lack of clear

P200 responses and increased amplitude of N100 responses in a group of tinnitus patients. A case study corroborated these findings and showed that evoked potentials were normalized during remission of tinnitus (Pantev et al., 1989). However, these promising findings were not replicated in two subsequent studies (Jacobson et al., 1991; Colding-Jørgensen et al., 1992). More recently, sophisticated measurement strategies have been utilized and selective attention has been manipulated, showing more promising results (Attias et al., 1996; Jacobson et al., 1996; Hoke et al., 1998; Norena et al., 1999). There are issues with the populations that have been used in these studies; for example, it can be argued that male army personnel, studied by Attias and co-workers, represent a distinct group from the mixed gender samples used in other studies. In a study by Kadner et al. (2002) auditory evoked potentials were recorded from eight tinnitus patients and 12 control subjects. Tone pips of 1000 Hz and 2000 Hz, as well as a tone matched to the frequency of the tinnitus (commonly around 4000 Hz), were presented at different intensities. Results showed a steeper response in the tinnitus group to the tinnitus frequency tone, and the authors hypothesized that the findings derived from lateral inhibition arising from neural activity in the 4000 Hz region. In another study by Walpurger et al. (2003) a fresh approach was taken when Hallam's habituation model was tested in a study with 10 tinnitus complainers and 12 non-complainers. Diminution of the N1 and P2 amplitudes of the evoked potentials were taken to measure habituation for consecutive trials. The results supported the habituation theory, with less distinct habituation in the group with more severe tinnitus.

In a study using magnetic source imaging, a magnetic encephalography technique that measures cortical responses by changes in magnetic fields rather than electrical responses, Mühlnickel et al. (1998) found evidence of cortical reorganization in response to auditory stimulation in a group of 10 tinnitus patients compared with 15 control subjects.

Positron emission tomography and related methods

Until recently, it was not possible to study deep brain functioning *in vivo*, but technological developments have dramatically changed this situation (Johnsrude et al., 2002). Tinnitus has recently been studied using single photon emission computed tomography (SPECT), positron emission tomography (PET) and functional magnetic resonance imaging (fMRI). The results are summarized in Table 7.1. For ease of interpretation, Brodmann's areas (BAs) are depicted in Figure 7.1.

SPECT is a technique which can be regarded as a predecessor of PET. Abraham Schulman and his colleagues found that the brain activity in two tinnitus patients was significantly different from normative data (Schulman,

Table 7.1 Overview of brain imaging studies of tinnitus

Study	Manipulations or study group(s)	Main results
SPECT		
Shulman et al. (1995)	Blood flow at rest compared with normative data. Two patients.	Significant regional abnormalities bilaterally in temporal, frontal, parietal, and hippocampal amygdala regions
Sataloff et al. (1996)	Blood flow at rest compared with normative data. Twelve patients.	Abnormal findings in 11 patients.
Staffen et al. (1999)	Lidocaine minus rest. Single case.	Lateralization between right and left auditory cortex decreased during lidocaine infusion.
Gardner et al. (2002)	Depressed patients with ($n=27$) or without ($n=18$) tinnitus.	Differences in right frontal lobe. In many patients activation of primary or secondary auditory cortex.
PET		
Arnold et al. (1996)	Ears plugged at rest. Eleven patients, 14 control subjects; one patient with fluctuating tinnitus.	Increased activity in primary auditory cortex (BA 41). Correspondence between complaints and PET.
Lockwood et al. (1998)	Oral facial movement or tone stimulation. Four tinnitus patients and six control subjects.	Activation in auditory cortex (BA 41). More widespread activation in patients, and activation of hippocampus.
Mirz et al. (1999a)	Masking versus rest. Lidocaine versus rest. Twelve patients.	Altered activity in middle frontal and middle temporal gyri and lateral and mesial posterior sites (BAs 41, 42, 21 and 8). Activation of right precuneus (BA 7) in lidocaine condition.
Giraud et al. (1999)	Gaze-evoked tinnitus. Four patients.	Activity in temporoparietal association auditory cortex, but not in primary auditory cortex. BAs 42, 21, 22, 7 and 8 activated.

Study	Subjects/method	Findings
Andersson et al. (2000b)	Lidocaine versus rest. One patient.	Increased rCBF in the left parieto-temporal auditory cortex, including the primary and secondary auditory cortex with a focus in the parietal cortex (BAs 39, 41, 42, 21 and 22). Activations were also found in right frontal paralimbic areas (BAs 47, 49 and 15).
Lockwood et al. (2001)	Gaze-evoked tinnitus. Eight tinnitus patients and seven control subjects.	Evidence for neural activity related to tinnitus seen in auditory lateral pontine tegmentum or auditory cortex.
Mirz et al. (2002)	Five cochlear implant patients with tinnitus. Tinnitus reduced by implant.	Activation of primary and secondary auditory cortex, limbic system and the precuneus (BA 7).
Reyes et al. (2002)	Lidocaine versus placebo. Ten tinnitus patients, seven control subjects.	Evidence for neural activity related to tinnitus seen in auditory lateral pontine tegmentum or auditory cortex. Less response to lidocaine than usually observed.
Andersson et al. (unpublished data)	Eight tinnitus patients. Silent counting backwards in steps of seven.	Reduced activity in auditory cortex bilaterally.
fMRI		
Cacace et al. (1996)	Gaze-evoked tinnitus ($n=2$) and one case with cutaneous-evoked tinnitus.	Abnormal foci of activity in the upper brainstem and frontal cortex.
Cacace et al. (1999)	Cutaneous-evoked tinnitus. Two patients.	Activation of temporoparietal junction.
Mirz et al. (1999b)	Masking versus rest. Eight patients.	Activation of superior and middle temporal gyri, BAs 21, 22, 37 and 39 (associative auditory cortex); BAs 7 and 40 (parietal lobes); BAs 8–10 and 44–45 (inferior frontal gyri); BAs 6, 9 and 31–32 (medial frontal and cingulate gyrus).
Melcher et al. (2000)	White noise stimulation. Four lateralized patients, three non-lateralized, compared with six control subjects.	Binaural noise produced abnormally low activation of the inferior colliculus in lateralized tinnitus.

BA = Brodmann's area.

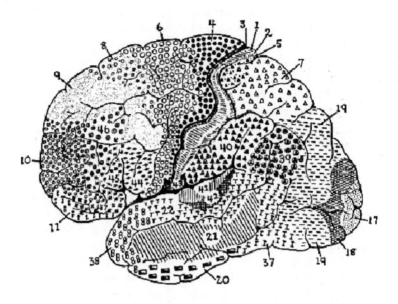

Figure 7.1 Brodmann's cytoarchitectural map of cortical areas of the brain.

1995). Sataloff et al. (1996) studied blood flow at rest in 12 patients, and when these data were compared with normative data as many as 11 patients were found to have abnormal findings. In a case study using lidocaine to temporarily abolish tinnitus, Staffen et al. (1999) compared differences in blood flow using SPECT between at rest and with tinnitus abolished by means of lidocaine. These workers found that the lateralization between left and right auditory cortex decreased following lidocaine infusion.

More recently, Gardner et al. (2002) used SPECT in a study of 45 patients with lifetime depression, of whom 27 had severe tinnitus. Decreased blood flow was found in the right frontal lobes (BA 45), left parietal lobes (BA 39), and left visual association cortices (BA 18) was found in the tinnitus group compared with the depressed patients without tinnitus. These workers also found that the proportion of tinnitus patients with pronounced rCBF (a measure of cortical blood flow) alterations in auditory cortex was increased compared with both a normal comparison sample and the depressed patients without tinnitus. It would have been interesting to know to what extent depressed versus non-depressed tinnitus patients differed in terms of cortical activity, but such a control group was not included.

PET is a more advanced technique that uses radio isotopes to obtain cross-sectional images of the body, and to highlight areas of increased metabolic activity. Commonly, the brain imaging application of PET consists of tracing blood flow by labelling isotopes of oxygen and other elements (Johnsrude et al., 2002). The use of PET in tinnitus research is increasingly popular, but is hampered by the costs and the need for intravenous injections of the tracer substance. Arnold et al. (1996) used PET to study 11 tinnitus patients at rest and compared the findings with a control group. The results showed an increase of cortical activity in primary auditory cortex in the tinnitus group. Interestingly, in one of the tinnitus subjects, tinnitus was weaker than usual at the time of the testing and the patient was therefore called in for a second session in which tinnitus was back at its usual level. These subjective reports of tinnitus were found to correspond to the PET data, with increased cortical activity in auditory cortex.

Lockwood et al. (1998) studied four patients who had tinnitus that they could modify by means of oral facial movements (jaw clenching). This is an interesting phenomenon that seems quite common among tinnitus patients in some studies (Pinchoff et al., 1998). This was a complex study, but the main finding was increased activity in the auditory cortex, and some evidence for the involvement of the hippocampus (a structure active in emotional processing) was also observed. Lockwood and colleagues also included a control group. Using auditory stimulation, their results showed that tinnitus patients displayed more widespread cortical activation than control subjects.

Mirz et al. (1999a) studied tinnitus suppression with PET using both lidocaine and masking by means of narrow-band noise. In total their 12 subjects underwent eight scans. In the lidocaine part of the study there were two non-responders. Results were analysed using a subtraction approach. These authors found a decrease in right middle frontal gyrus and middle temporal gyri (BA 21) activity following lidocaine administration. Interestingly, the right precuneus was also activated. In a masking versus baseline condition, the results showed that all 12 subjects masked their tinnitus and a decrease in primary auditory cortex activity was found, extending into associate areas. This study has been questioned because of a suspected lack of statistical significance (Reyes et al., 2002; Cacace, 2003).

Giraud et al. (1999) studied four patients with gaze-evoked tinnitus that had developed after unilateral vestibular schwannoma surgery. Changes in eye gaze resulted in activation of temporoparietal association auditory cortex (BA 42, 21 and 22), but not in the primary auditory cortex. The precuneus (BA 7) was also activated with increased tinnitus.

Andersson et al. (2000b) reported a case in which lidocaine was used effectively to inhibit tinnitus. The brain activity associated with tinnitus included the left primary, secondary and integrative auditory brain areas (Figure 7.2), as well as right paralimbic areas, which are thought to be involved in processing negative feelings. Increased activity in association with tinnitus was also found in the left parietal cortex (precuneus, BA 7).

Lockwood et al. (2001) also used PET to study gaze-evoked tinnitus in eight patients and included a control group consisting of seven age- and gender-matched subjects. Results showed activation of auditory lateral pontine tegmentum or auditory cortex. More detailed tables of their data

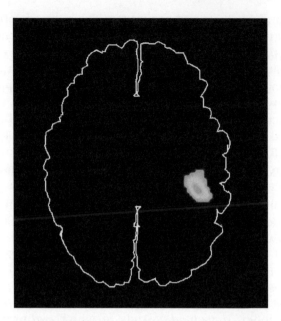

Figure 7.2 PET images of tinnitus-related brain activity. The figure describes activation in the tinnitus–lidocaine contrast (Andersson et al., 2000). Increased activity is found in primary and secondary auditory cortex. (Reprinted by permission of the publisher Taylor & Francis.)

with Brodmann areas revealed that activation of secondary auditory cortex structures were evident, as was found by Giraud et al. (1999).

In the most recent lidocaine study, Reyes et al. (2002) studied 10 subjects and, surprisingly, found that only five patients had a decrease in their tinnitus, whereas four patients reported an increase. One patient had no change. Most important, given the well-known placebo effect, these authors included a lidocaine placebo condition. The results showed that increase of tinnitus was associated with activity in the secondary auditory cortex of the right hemisphere (BA 21). It would have been interesting to see the activation caused by the placebo minus baseline condition, but these data were not reported.

In an innovative study, Mirz et al. (2002) reported an experiment in which five cochlear implant patients with tinnitus were studied. All had in common the experience that tinnitus was totally suppressed by turning on the implant. Subtraction analyses showed that primary and secondary auditory cortex structures were activated during tinnitus, but also the parahippocampal gyrus (BA 35) on the right side, and the precuneus on the right side.

Andersson and co-workers (unpublished data) studied eight patients and found that silent backwards counting (serial sevens test) lead to a decrease in neural activity in the auditory cortex (BAs 41, 42 and 22), as well as perceived decrease of tinnitus loudness and annoyance. The reduced cortical activity can be seen as a replication of what has been found in previous studies on normal subjects (Ghatan et al., 1996; Ghatan et al., 1998). It is worth noting that primary auditory cortex was more clearly involved than in the previous studies on normal subjects. Unfortunately, a control group of subjects without tinnitus was not included in the study.

fMRI is a specialized form of MRI scanning that measures blood flow in tissues. Increased blood flow is used to imply increased activity within the tissue. Unlike PET scanning, this does not require the use of potentially hazardous radioactive isotopes in tinnitus research. However, fMRI scanning produces noise up to 130 dB, which limits its usefulness in auditory research. Also, although subjects undergoing such scans can wear noise-attenuating devices, some patients with tinnitus and hyperacusis are deterred by the noise.

Cacace et al. (1996) used fMRI in two patients with gaze-evoked tinnitus and found signs of abnormal activity in the upper brainstem and in the frontal cortex. In a later study of two patients with cutaneous-evoked tinnitus (Cacace, 1999), activation of the temporoparietal junction was found.

Mirz et al. (1999b) presented a study in which eight patients were investigated with fMRI at rest and while they were having their tinnitus masked. The results showed activation of associative auditory cortex (BAs 21, 22, 37 and 39), the parietal lobes (BAs 7 and 40), inferior frontal gyri, and medial frontal and cingulate gyri (BAs 6, 9 and 31–32).

Melcher et al. (2000) managed to use a quieter fMRI method by focusing on a restricted area of the brain. Using a complex design, four patients with lateralized tinnitus were compared with three with non-lateralized tinnitus and six control subjects, of whom several also had tinnitus: the use of such a control group is somewhat perplexing. As in the study by Mirz et al. (1999b), a masking approach was used. The main finding was that binaural noise produced abnormally low activation of the inferior colliculus in patients with lateralized tinnitus. The inferior colliculus has been suggested to be of significance in tinnitus (Gerken, 1996) given its role in lateral inhibition.

Measures of neural activity associated with tinnitus

As described in Chapter 3, research into mechanisms of tinnitus has involved subjecting animals to agents that induce tinnitus in humans (specifically noise and salycilate), and recording changes in neural activity that might represent tinnitus. These recording techniques have not been widely applied to humans, however. Martin (1995) described spectral average recordings from the cochlear nerve of 14 human adult patients undergoing cerebellopontine angle surgery. In 12 patients with tinnitus, a prominent peak in the spectral average near 200 Hz was reported.

Integrating the findings and future directions

Findings from brain imaging studies attest that tinnitus can be measured objectively. The findings are not consistent, but it is clear that tinnitus affects brain areas related to hearing and processing of sounds, but also that some involvement of the brain's emotional and attentional systems might be involved (e.g. amygdala). It is interesting to note that it is often the case that secondary rather than primary auditory cortex has been activated in several imaging studies. Of note, Mirz et al. (1999c) found that an interrupted stream of tones activated the secondary auditory associative cortex, whereas a tone predictably activated the primary cortex. Tinnitus has often been explained in terms of increased firing rates (Rauschecker, 1999), but data from imaging studies perhaps suggest the opposite of a slower firing rate, leading the brain to interpret intermittent streams of neural information as a tone.

In a novel study, Mirz et al. (2000) used PET and studied 12 healthy subjects to whom they presented 'tinnitus sounds' derived from actual tinnitus matching data. The results showed that the tinnitus sounds lead to activation of primary (BA 41) and right associative auditory cortex (BAs 21 and 22) and limbic structures such as the amygdala or parahippocampal gyrus and hippocampus.

Various imaging studies have found that the precuneus (BA 7) is activated in tinnitus patients, suggesting that it is an important area in the perception of tinnitus. Interestingly, Blood et al. (1999) found that the degree of dissonance in musical passages correlated with increased activity in BA 7 on the right side. This area has also been related to attentional mechanisms, and to auditory hallucinations (Shergill et al., 2000). Moreover, increased activity in the precuneus, has been found in association with cognitive tasks (Ghatan et al., 1998; Zatorre and Binder, 2000).

Imaging tinnitus is an emergent field, and several important research issues remain to be investigated. Manipulation of emotion is a possible area for further work given that both the neurophysiological and the psychological models emphasize this aspect of tinnitus experience. Another possible area to explore is the outcome of habituation-based treatments to try to ascertain objective evidence of their efficacy – or otherwise. Imaging techniques could also be used to evaluate other treatment modalities. An example of the emergence of such studies is a study by Langguth et al. (2003), in which a single patient was given low-frequency repetitive transcranial magnetic stimulation. The effects were evaluated in a single-blind, sham-controlled, crossover manner, followed by a four-week open treatment. After active stimulation there was a decrease in tinnitus which was paralleled by altered cortical excitability. Clearly, these findings need to be replicated in a larger setting with more participants, a fact that was acknowledged by the authors. Most imaging studies on tinnitus fail to account for possible co-morbid psychiatric conditions. The main exception is the study by Gardner et al. (2002), in which patients with concurrent tinnitus and depression were included. In future imaging studies it would be interesting to investigate the differences between distressed versus non-distressed tinnitus patients, as it is possible that cortical activation, in particular cortical reorganization, might differ in relation to levels of distress.

Despite the encouraging work concerning tinnitus imaging, some workers have sounded notes of caution. Current imaging techniques have been criticized with suggestions that they might not be sensitive enough to capture the relevant brain mechanisms involved in tinnitus (Johnsrude et al., 2002).

Summary

Researchers and clinicians have long suspected that tinnitus involves certain specific areas of the brain, in particular those that subserve the perception and amplification of the experience (Minton, 1923). There are indications that tinnitus patients' reaction times differ from control subjects without tinnitus: tinnitus patients seem to display faster reaction time to sounds at the tinnitus frequency (Goodwin and Johnson, 1980a, 1980b; Nieschalk et al., 1998). Additional data have been collected by use of evoked response audiometry. In a few studies the results have not been conclusive (Barnea et al., 1990; McKee and Stephens, 1992; Attias et al., 1996), but other studies have indicated that early as well as later latency waves are affected in tinnitus (Maurizi et al., 1985; Ikner and Hassen, 1990; Rosenhall and Axelsson, 1995). It is possible that sample characteristics of the studies, such as differences of the test populations, may explain these contradictory findings. Imaging techniques have produced some interesting results – with the overall message that auditory areas of the brain show increased activity in tinnitus patients. There are some inconsistencies in the data from imaging studies but, despite this, it remains an exciting area of tinnitus research.

Chapter 8
Self-report and interview measures of tinnitus severity and impact

As stated previously, there are no objective ways to determine the severity of tinnitus. Whilst there are indeed associations between the degree of hearing loss and tinnitus annoyance, audiometric data provide little information about tinnitus distress in individual cases. In many ways, what distinguishes mild from severe tinnitus is difficult to establish, apart from variations in subjective ratings of intrusiveness and loudness. Moreover, attempts to determine the handicap caused by tinnitus using the characteristics of the tinnitus itself, such as loudness, pitch and character, have not proved helpful to date. Therefore, it is necessary to carefully interview the patient to get an idea of the level of distress associated with tinnitus. This is crucial as psychological complaints are of major importance in determining the severity of tinnitus.

In line with the difficulties associated with measuring tinnitus (see Chapter 6), no consensus has been reached regarding its classification, although several schemes have been proposed (Douek, 1981; Nodar, 1996; Holgers et al., 2000) that have included guidelines on how to measure severity. In addition, there have been several alternative suggestions in terms of cut-off scores on questionnaire measures (e.g. McCombe et al., 2001), but it is fair to say already at the outset of this chapter that there is no consensus on how severity of tinnitus should best be assessed.

Dauman and Tyler (1992) proposed a system involving several classifications (see Table 8.1). These workers distinguished between normal and pathological tinnitus, the former being a sensation experienced sometimes by most people (Heller and Bergman 1953) and the latter being defined by its prolonged nature (more than five minutes every week) and its association with hearing loss. Dauman and Tyler (1992) classified tinnitus by its severity, duration, site of origin and aetiology. Of particular interest is the classification of tinnitus severity into acceptable and unacceptable. However, exactly how unacceptable tinnitus was defined was not described, although this was probably intended to be based on an interview with the patient.

Table 8.1 Dauman and Tyler's (1992) classification system of tinnitus

Pathology	Severity	Duration	Site of origin	Aetiology
Normal	Acceptable	Temporary	Middle ear	Noise-induced
Pathological	Unacceptable	Permanent	Peripheral neural	Ménière's disease
				Ototoxicity
			Central neural	Presbyacusis
				Unknown
				aetiology

Adapted from Davis and Rafaie (2000).

Klockhoff and Lindblom (1967) devised a system for the determination of tinnitus severity and distress that has been used in Sweden (following slight modification by Scott et al., 1990). The grading system is presented in Table 8.2, and it can be regarded as a mixture of the perceptual and experiential aspects of tinnitus. Andersson et al. (1999) reported data from a study that included a sub-sample of 39 patients for whom tinnitus grading had been assessed both by a clinical psychologist and an ENT physician. A significant correlation was found between the two forms of assessment (Rho = 0.80; p = 0.0001]. Further, similar proportions of patients were assessed as grade I (5.1%), grade II (64.1%) and grade III (30.8%) by the physician when comparing the ratings conducted by the clinical psychologist (4.2%, 57.5% and 38.3%, respectively). A set of discriminant analyses was conducted on the data set to investigate variables discriminating between tinnitus of grades II and III. This resulted in a final model that included pitch, minimal masking level, tolerance in relation to onset and avoidance of situations because of tinnitus. This model correctly classified 73% of the subjects into the two levels of distress (grades II and III).

Table 8.2 Klockhoff and Lindblom (1967) and Scott et al. (1990)

Grade I	Tinnitus is audible only in silent environments
Grade II	Tinnitus is audible only in ordinary acoustic environments, but masked by loud environmental sounds; it can disturb going to sleep, but not sleep in general
Grade III	Tinnitus is audible in all acoustic environments, disturbs going to sleep, can disturb sleep in general, and is a dominating problem that affects quality of life

In comparison, the Dauman and Tyler (1992) system is more comprehensive, but the Klockhoff and Lindblom (1967) system does have the advantage of providing a single global rating of the severity of tinnitus, and it is used as such in current clinical practice. The grading system has been used in research studies, and a common observation is that among patients seeking help for hearing loss (with co-morbid tinnitus), and in patients operated on for vestibular schwannoma, relatively few have grade III tinnitus (6–14 %) (Lindberg et al., 1984; Andersson et al., 1997). Lindberg et al. (1984) reported that 35% of their tinnitus sample of hearing aid centre clients had tinnitus of grade I and 51% had tinnitus of grade II. Tinnitus of grade III appears to be rare in the general population, but the relative prevalence of tinnitus of grades I and II is not known.

Structured interviews

There are few reports on the use of structured interviews with tinnitus patients. Most clinicians follow an interview protocol that gives a framework of topics to discuss at the first consultation but few have evaluated if the questions used are appropriate. Lindberg and Scott developed a structured interview, which was later revised (Andersson et al., 1999). The interview is conducted after audiological and medical examinations. The questions are summarized in Table 8.3. Other researchers have developed similar approaches (Hiller and Goebel, 1999). The structured interview needs to be complemented with questionnaire data and is best regarded in relation to findings from audiological tests.

Tinnitus self-report measures

Self-report measures are increasingly used in both the management of tinnitus patients and in tinnitus research. With the advent of evidence-based medicine, the use of clear and robust outcome measures is of great importance. In particular, controversies about the efficacies of treatment methods will not be resolved until those efficacies can be determined in a manner that allows direct comparison.

Visual analogue scales

Daily diaries provide an indispensable tool both in research and in practice. It is common for tinnitus to fluctuate, and on occasion patients have difficulty identifying reasons for such fluctuations. Diaries can supply the answer in many cases. Daily diaries need to be easily comprehended and unobtrusive while still providing usable data. One alternative, which is commonly used in pain management, is the visual analogue scale (VAS). This is simply a straight line, the end anchors of which are labelled as the extreme boundaries of the sensation, feeling or response being measured (Wewers and Lowe, 1990). Sometimes the rating on a VAS is collected on single occasions and not for a

Table 8.3 Summary of the questions asked in structured tinnitus interview

1	Background data (age, etc.)
2	Hearing loss and use of hearing aid (including effects on tinnitus)
3	Tinnitus localization
4	Tinnitus primary character, including descriptors of tinnitus
5	Duration of tinnitus
6	Event(s) associated with onset of tinnitus (e.g. trauma)
7	Tinnitus grading (Klockhoff and Lindblom, 1967)
8	Variation in tinnitus loudness
9	Attention directed towards tinnitus during an ordinary day
10	Most problematic situations associated with tinnitus
11	Time of the day most problematic
12	Possibility to do something to lessen the problems with tinnitus
13	Possibility to change the loudness of tinnitus
14	Situations when tinnitus is less problematic
15	Avoidance of situations and activities because of tinnitus
16	Psychological consequences of tinnitus, including irritation, depression, anxiety and concentration difficulties
17	Sleep problems (hours sleep per night, sleep onset latency, awakenings during the night, time awake in the morning)
18	Influence of background sounds or noises on tinnitus
19	Masking of tinnitus by background sounds
20	Noise sensitivity, including hyperacusis
21	Influence of stress and fatigue
22	Influence of weather
23	Medication or other causes than tinnitus and their effects on tinnitus
24	Use of caffeine and its effects on tinnitus
25	Alcohol use and effects on tinnitus
26	Tobacco use (cigarette and snuff) and effects on tinnitus
27	Role of relatives or spouse when coping with tinnitus
28	Major or minor change of tinnitus characteristics since onset
29	Tolerance of tinnitus in relation to onset (e.g. much better or much worse)
30	Earlier or ongoing treatments for tinnitus and hearing loss (including counselling)
31	Perceived cause of tinnitus
32	Problems with headache
33	Dizziness or unsteadiness
34	Muscular tension (in face, jaws or shoulders)
35	Earlier or ongoing psychiatric consultations or treatments
36	Attitude towards tinnitus
37	Attitude towards referral to psychologist
38	Presentation of a cognitive–behavioural model of tinnitus annoyance and check for acceptance of the model and the approach to treatment (including time investment, not a cure, etc.

Based on Andersson (2001).

series of days (or hours). It is important to note that one single rating on a VAS is not very reliable and the strength of the method lies in the aggregation of several measurements (e.g. a weekly average of tinnitus annoyance). Although the VAS has been recommended for use in tinnitus research (Axelsson et al., 1993), it is not clear how commonly it is used in clinical practice. An example of a VAS is given in Figure 8.1.

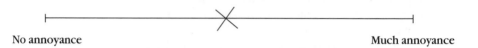

No annoyance   Much annoyance

Figure 8.1 A visual analogue scale.

Tinnitus-specific questionnaires

For clinical use a questionnaire must be brief and easy to interpret. It should also be appropriate and understandable to the patient and the results should be easy to feed back in the consulting room. There are several instruments available, and although a comparative assessment is difficult many of the items included in the questionnaires are often rather similar (for reviews *see* Tyler, 1993; Noble, 2000; Holgers and Barrenäs, 2003). Examples of items included in two common questionnaires are given in Table 8.4.

Table 8.4 Examples of items in the Tinnitus Reaction Questionnaire and the Tinnitus Handicap Inventory

Tinnitus Reaction Questionnaire (Wilson et al., 1991)

    My tinnitus has made me unhappy
    My tinnitus has 'driven me crazy'
    My tinnitus has lead me to avoid noisy situations
    My tinnitus has interfered with my ability to work

Tinnitus Handicap Inventory (Newman et al., 1996)

    Because of your tinnitus is it difficult for you to concentrate?
    Do you complain a great deal about your tinnitus?
    Do you feel that you have no control over your tinnitus?
    Does your tinnitus make you feel insecure?

Similar factors tend to become evident when conducting factor analyses, reflecting the fact that a substantial overlap exists in questionnaire wording of items and content. A list of questionnaires is presented in Table 8.5.

Table 8.5 Overview of tinnitus self-report inventories

Title	Number of items and factors	Psychometrics
Tinnitus Questionnaire (Hallam, 1996a)	52 items, five factors	$\alpha = 0.91$ for total scale, for subscales $\alpha = 0.76$ to $\alpha = 0.94$
Tinnitus Handicap Questionnaire (Kuk et al., 1990)	27 items, three factors	$\alpha = 0.93$ for total scale
Tinnitus Severity Scale (Sweetow and Levy, 1990)	15 items	Alpha not reported
Tinnitus Reaction Questionnaire (Wilson et al., 1991)	26 items, four factors	$\alpha = 0.96$ and a test–retest correlation of $r = 0.88$
Subjective Tinnitus Severity Scale (Halford and Anderson, 1991a)	16 items	$\alpha = 0.84$
Tinnitus Handicap/Support Scale (Erlandsson et al., 1992)	28 items, three factors	Alpha not reported
Tinnitus Handicap Inventory (Newman et al., 1996)	25 items, three scales	$\alpha = 0.93$ for total scale

One of the first questionnaires developed specifically for the assessment of tinnitus complaints, was the 'Tinnitus Questionnaire' (Hallam, 1996a), which exists in two versions. The questionnaire was first called the 'Tinnitus Effects Questionnaire', but this was later shortened to the 'Tinnitus Questionnaire'. The full Tinnitus Questionnaire contains 52 items and covers sleep, emotional disturbances, audiological or perceptual difficulties and intrusiveness. In a factor analysis of an earlier 40-item version, Hallam et al. (1988) extracted three factors: sleep disturbance; emotional disturbances; and audiological or perceptual disturbances. Hiller and Goebel (1992) factor-analysed the 52-item version and found a five-factor solution. In addition to Hallam's factors these authors added a factor called 'intrusiveness' and one entitled 'somatic complaints'. The intrusiveness factor was also noted in an earlier study by Jakes et al. (1985). There is also a briefer 33-item version of the Tinnitus Questionnaire, for which Hallam (1989) proposed six factors: helplessness; capacity for rest and relaxation; acceptability of change; emotional effects and related beliefs; hearing speech and sounds; and ability to ignore. This ordering of items into subscales was not, however, derived from empirical analysis.

The Tinnitus Reaction Questionnaire was developed by Wilson and co-workers (1991) and has been used in several research studies and in different languages (e.g. English, German, French and Swedish). It has also been validated for Internet use (Andersson et al., 2003b). The Tinnitus Reaction Questionnaire was designed specifically to measure distress – such as tension, depression and anger – that may be related to tinnitus. It has repeatedly been found to generate good psychometric properties. A principal components analysis suggested four factors, labelled 'general distress', 'interference', 'severity' and 'avoidance'. Meric et al. (2000) refrained from factor-analysing the French version, assuming a priori the factorial structure to be extant. However, given the high internal consistency found, and on the basis of factor analyses of the Swedish version of the Tinnitus Reaction Questionnaire, it is very likely that the scale contains only one reliable factor from a statistical point of view. In other words, there is a substantial overlap in how patients respond to the items in the Tinnitus Reaction Questionnaire.

The Tinnitus Handicap Questionnaire was developed by Kuk et al. (1990), informed by their previous research on open-ended questions. The questionnaire was properly analysed by means of principal components factor analysis, which resulted in three factors, with the first two being particularly noteworthy. The first reflected physical, emotional and social consequences of tinnitus, and the second factor reflected hearing. The last factor was seen as mirroring patients' views on tinnitus. Together they explained 57.6% of the variance, but as has been seen in subsequent factor analyses of other tinnitus questionnaires, the first factor explained the majority of the variance (42.6%). This suggests that a basic overarching annoyance factor is involved. This questionnaire has not been widely used in research, but was recently validated for a French population (Bouscau-Faure et al., 2003). However, Goebel and Hiller (1999) raised some concerns over test construction and composition of the scales.

The Tinnitus Severity Scale (Sweetow and Levy, 1990) is a small scale with 15 items, but was developed with the aim of covering several aspects with few items. Brevity is often advantageous in clinical settings, rendering this scale attractive in some settings. However, the published report did not include enough information to assess the suitability of the scale from a psychometric point of view.

Another questionnaire, the Subjective Tinnitus Severity Scale (Halford and Anderson, 1991a) was developed with items again reflecting the annoyance/intrusion dimension of tinnitus. In another report (Halford and Anderson, 1991b), the authors found the scale correlated with measures of anxiety and depression, a common finding in the literature.

A Swedish research group developed a Tinnitus Handicap/Support Scale (Erlandsson et al., 1992). This scale includes several important dimensions, such as social support, and seems to possess adequate psychometric properties. Unfortunately, this scale has not been translated into any other language.

The Tinnitus Handicap Inventory (Newman et al., 1996) is widely used internationally in the clinical context to assess tinnitus-related self-reported handicap and to report treatment outcomes (Newman et al., 1998; Rosenberg et al., 1998; McCombe et al. 2001). Moreover, high convergent validity with other measures of tinnitus distress, specifically with the Tinnitus Questionnaire (Hallam, 1996a), have been reported (Baguley et al., 2000). The Tinnitus Handicap Inventory has been translated into Danish (Zachariae et al., 2000) and Spanish (Herraiz et al., 2001). Newman et al. (1996), in the original presentation of the Tinnitus Handicap Inventory, suggested a three-component model for the Tinnitus Handicap Inventory, naming the factors 'Emotional', 'Functional' and 'Catastrophic'. However, the factor structure of the scale was not initially reported. Factor analysis of the sub-scales of the Tinnitus Handicap Inventory has later been reported for the Danish translation (Zachariae et al., 2000). In this study an exploratory factor analysis (incorrectly presented as a confirmatory factor analysis) demonstrated that a three-factor solution could be derived, but the factors were not identical to the ones suggested a priori by Newman et al. (1996). In a recent factor analysis it was found to contain only one factor and not the three suggested in the original paper (Baguley and Andersson, 2003).

A set of targeted tinnitus questionnaires has been developed. For example, an Australian research group has devised a Tinnitus Coping Strategy Questionnaire (Henry and Wilson, 1995). It contains 33 items dealing with the cognitive and behavioural strategies used to cope with tinnitus. Two ratings are made for each item, one dealing with frequency of usage and the other dealing with derived benefit. The questionnaire is very much inspired by the Coping Strategy Questionnaire used in pain research (Rosentiel and Keefe, 1983). The Tinnitus Coping Strategy Questionnaire is reported to have excellent psychometric properties (Chronbach's α = 0.88) for each of the two summary scales (e.g. Frequency and Benefit). There is yet another questionnaire targeted towards coping with tinnitus, the Tinnitus Coping Style Questionnaire (Budd and Pugh, 1996a, 1996b). It includes 40 items, and has been factor-analysed into two stable factors called 'maladaptive' and 'effective' coping styles. Wilson and Henry (1998) have also developed a Tinnitus Cognitions Questionnaire and have used it in outcome research (Henry and Wilson, 1998).

Open-ended approaches

Stephens and co-workers suggested an alternative approach to questionnaire assessment involving open-ended questions that are classified and quantified. It has been suggested that treatment effects may be more easily detected by open-ended questions than by structured questionnaires, for example the

Tinnitus Questionnaire (Sadlier and Stephens, 1995). This method could potentially be useful in the study of tinnitus, but may also result in inconsistencies. For example, using the open-ended approach, Tyler and Baker (1983) reported that 33% of the tinnitus patients had concentration problems. Sanchez and Stephens (1997) found a slightly lower percentage of 22% reporting concentration problems in response to the question 'Make a list of the difficulties you have as a result of your tinnitus.' However, when confronted with the question in either a structured interview (Andersson and Lyttkens, 1999) or in a questionnaire (Andersson et al., 2001) 70% and 78%, respectively, of tinnitus patients reported that they had concentration problems. Discrepancies between open-ended versus closed question sets, with open-ended questions yielding lower frequencies, has been observed in other studies (Schwartz, 1999). Although open-ended questions are certainly valid they are not necessarily reliable.

Other useful self-report instruments

Proper multidisciplinary management of tinnitus patients often requires the assessment of related aspects, which can be even more disabling than tinnitus. One such example is the experience of hearing loss, for which several questionnaires have been developed and validated (Andersson et al., 1995a; Ringdahl et al., 1998). Noble (1998) provides a comprehensive review of these measures. Self-report measures of hearing disability and handicap may provide useful information about hearing dysfunction. This can be of particular importance when it is possible to fit a hearing aid to improve communication, but it can also be the case that communication strategies (e.g. hearing tactics) are lacking and need to be targeted in rehabilitation.

Given the increased recognition of psychological factors when dealing with tinnitus, the use of validated measures of depression and anxiety can be useful, both when planning and evaluating the treatment. One alternative is the Hospital Anxiety and Depression Scale (Zigmond and Snaith, 1983), which includes only 14 items (response scale 0–3). One advantage with the Hospital Anxiety and Depression Scale is that it has been developed for use with somatic patients and hence controls for complaints better explained by the somatic problem (Bjelland et al., 2002). Zigmond and Snaith (1983) recommended a cut-off score for 'cases' of 11 or more on each of the two sub-scales as being indicative of being 'cases' of either anxiety or depression. Other cut-off scores have been suggested; for example, eight on each of the sub-scales (Bjelland et al., 2002). It needs to be made clear that the Hospital Anxiety and Depression Scale, and any other self-report inventory for that matter, is not a substitute for a proper psychiatric assessment, which should be requested in difficult cases.

Insomnia can be assessed with the Insomnia Severity Index (Bastien et al., 2001). This is a seven-item questionnaire suitable for detecting changes in perceived sleep difficulties (Bastien et al., 2001). Each item is scored on an 0–4 Likert-type scale and a sum is calculated. Bastien et al. (2001) reported an internal consistency of $\alpha = 0.74$.

Tinnitus patients often report cognitive failures. The Cognitive Failures Questionnaire (Broadbent et al., 1982) is a self-report inventory for the assessment of common everyday errors regarding perception, memory and motor function. It contains 25 items and has adequate psychometric properties. It has also been used with tinnitus patients (McKenna, 1997).

There are several questionnaires available for the assessment of quality of life. Perhaps the most common is the Short Form 36 (SF-36) (Ware, 1993), which measures mobility and physical function, and for which normative data are published. The SF-36 has also been used in studies of tinnitus (Wilson et al., 2002). Although quality of life measures may be useful for research, they do not add much in clinical practice. El Rafaie et al. (1999) reported data on a newly developed Quality of Family Life Questionnaire, but this questionnaire has not yet been widely used.

How tinnitus affects the family and primary relations surrounding the individual with tinnitus is not well understood. Granqvist et al. (2001) used a tinnitus-adapted version of the Family Support Scale of the West Haven–Yale Multidimensional Pain Inventory (Kerns et al., 1985) for the purpose of measuring perceptions of family members' responses to the individual with tinnitus (see also Sullivan et al., 1994). This measure is not widely used.

Discussion

The assessment of tinnitus severity and impact is very much dependent on valid and reliable self-report instruments. To date, there has been no consensus about which to use in the research community or in clinics worldwide. Unfortunately, this means that neither research data nor audit of clinical activities can be compared. Goebel and Hiller (1999) did a critical comparison of the nine scientifically relevant and tinnitus-specific questionnaires that were then in existence worldwide. They recommended Hallam's Tinnitus Questionnaire, but unfortunately this measure is not widely known in the audiological community. Instead, the Tinnitus Handicap Inventory represents an alternative that could serve as an initial step towards consensus across communities (Surr et al., 1999). However, the Tinnitus Handicap Inventory largely measures psychological reactions towards tinnitus, neglecting other areas. Tyler (1993) concluded the comparative efficacy of the tinnitus specific scales is yet to be reported (but see Goebel and Hiller, 1999). In addition there are aspects not covered in the existing scales. Such aspects include common co-morbid problems such as hyperacusis, matters relating to avoidance of either noisy environments or silence and their direct effects on the experience of tinnitus. Other neglected factors include the sound characteristics of tinnitus and masking properties of environmental sound.

Summary

Although several classification schemes have been used in the literature, there remains a need to further develop a classification of tinnitus, and in particular to assess the effects of tinnitus on general well-being and quality of life. In order to get an idea of the disability caused by tinnitus, reliable and valid instruments are needed. It might be useful to apply the World Health Organization definition of impairment, disability and handicap (WHO, 1980), but also the recent International Classification of Functioning, Disability and Health (ICF) redefinition of 'body functions and structure; activities, participation, and contextual factors' (WHO, 2001). Noble (1998) suggested that interference with hearing functions represents the disability component of tinnitus, and that the emotional, health and sleep problems reflect the handicap component. At present there are several instruments devoted to the assessment of tinnitus, but as yet there is no self-report inventory that includes more than a fraction of the relevant aspects of tinnitus severity. For example, it is hard to understand why the commonly reported symptom of insomnia is seldom covered, but also why no measure even attempts to cover the important aspect of tinnitus maskability by environmental or background sounds.

Chapter 9
Consequences and moderating factors

For many years it has been recognized that tinnitus is associated with a range of problems (Fowler, 1948).Whilst there are still many unanswered questions, today our understanding of the nature and complexity of tinnitus has become more sophisticated. Among the first in the modern era to highlight this complexity were Tyler and Baker (1983), who found that tinnitus is associated with multiple symptoms in most people and that many of these symptoms were not primarily aural in nature. Since then others have added to this tapestry of tinnitus complaint. It is now agreed that the most common problems associated with tinnitus are sleep disturbance, emotional disturbance and concentration problems, as well as auditory perceptual disorders such as interference with hearing or increased sensitivity to noise (Hallam et al., 1988). Evidence is now emerging that children's experiences of tinnitus parallel those of adults, but are expressed in age-appropriate terms; sleep disturbance seems to be the main issue in children (Kentish et al., 2000). It is important to recognize the most common non-auditory consequences of tinnitus and to understand why some people but not others experience these effects.

Emotion and psychiatric state

The link between tinnitus and emotional distress has been investigated in several studies (Wood et al., 1983; Stephens and Hallam, 1985; Harrop-Griffiths et al., 1987; Simpson et al., 1988; Kirsch et al., 1989; Collet et al., 1990; Halford and Anderson, 1991b; McKenna et al., 1991; Scott and Lindberg, 2000). McKenna et al. (1991) reported that 45% of those whose main complaint was tinnitus showed signs of significant psychological disturbance. The idea that tinnitus might lead to psychological disturbance may seem self-evident. The onset of tinnitus constitutes a change in a person's life, and it may represent a number of losses, such as loss of silence or loss of control over an aspect of life. It is therefore likely that the person experiencing this change will also experience some sort of adjustment reaction to it. Within this type of reaction the person may suffer a variety of distressing states, such as disbelief, anger, anxiety and depression. These moods should pass over a period of weeks or a few months as the adjustment takes place. When the distress persists beyond this time and becomes more stable (e.g. more clearly depression rather than changing moods) then a mood disorder becomes established. In cognitive behavioural terms this happens when rational beliefs, such as 'I shall never hear silence again . . .' become overgeneralized, for example, '. . . therefore I shall never be happy again'. It must be remembered, however, that most studies on the emotional consequences of tinnitus have been conducted on highly selected samples of patients with severe tinnitus distress (Briner et al., 1990) and not all studies have found high levels of distress among tinnitus patients. Kirsch et al. (1989) and Wilson et al. (1991), using larger samples, revealed mean scores on self report measures of emotional state within the range of mild mood disturbance.

Most studies in this area have used questionnaire measures such as the General Health Questionnaire (Goldberg, 1978) or the Beck Depression Inventory (Beck et al., 1961) to assess psychological problems. Rather than relying just on questionnaire measures, some studies have assessed tinnitus patients' psychological state using formal psychiatric diagnostic methods (American Psychiatric Association, 1994). For example, Simpson et al. (1988) found that that a high proportion (63%) of tinnitus sufferers could be classified as psychiatrically disturbed or as having a had mood disorder (46%) as assessed by the Structured Interview for the *Diagnostic and Statistical Manual of Mental Disorders* (DSM-III-R) (First et al., 1997). The structured interview was also employed in a study by Sullivan et al. (1988). These researchers also found that a high proportion (78%) of their sample of tinnitus patients had experienced one or more episodes of major depression in their lifetime compared with the experiences of a control group (21%). Sullivan et al. (1988) also found that 60% of tinnitus patients had a major depression at the time of interview compared with 7% of the control group. Hiller and Goebel (1992b) found that 26 of 27 tinnitus patients fulfilled the DSM-III-R criteria for at least one lifetime diagnosis. Russo et al. (1994) used the DSM-IV to estimate the prevalence of psychiatric disorder among 88 tinnitus patients. No specific figures were provided for separate diagnoses, but it was reported that the average number of current and past diagnoses were 0.7 and 0.6, respectively. Zöger et al. (2001) studied a group of 82 tinnitus patients using DSM-IV diagnostic criteria. Their results showed that 62% of the patients had signs of lifetime depressive illness and that 39% had an ongoing depression. Current anxiety disorders (one or more) were found in 45% of patients, but of these a majority had co-morbid depression (69%). A high prevalence of psychiatric disorder (77% of cases) was also found among tinnitus patients in an Italian audiology clinic (Marciano et al., 2003). Using a novel approach, the Internet has recently been used to generate probable psychiatric diagnoses (Andersson et al., 2004). In that study, the World

Health Organization Composite International Diagnostic Interview – Short Form (CIDI-SF) (Kessler et al., 1998) was administered in a computerized Internet-based version to a self-selected sample of tinnitus patients ($n = 48$). Using the cut-off for 'probable case' (12-month prevalence), 69% of the tinnitus patients fulfilled the criteria for depression.

All these studies have in common that a remarkably high percentage of psychiatric disturbances has been found, well above what is found in the general population. However, in all studies it is very likely that selected sample groups have been studied that are not representative of the whole tinnitus population. Therefore, Andersson et al. replicated the study by Zöger et al. (2001) with a series of consecutive patients seen by an audiological physician in regular clinic. No selection was made on the basis of severity of tinnitus or degree of hearing impairment. In total 81 patients were interviewed with the SCID and they also completed tinnitus-related questionnaires, the Hospital Anxiety and Depression Scale, and a measure of sleep disturbance. Results showed a point prevalence of 14% for mood disorders and 31% for anxiety disorders. The lifetime prevalences were 42% for mood disorders and 38% for anxiety disorders. Concerning the onset of each disorder it was found that, for 56% of the patients, the first episode of mood disorder preceded the tinnitus onset; for 23.5% of patients, tinnitus preceded the mood disorder and for 20.5% of patients the onset of tinnitus and depression was simultaneous. Patients with an ongoing mood disorder had significantly higher scores on all self-report questionnaires (including tinnitus distress as measured by the Tinnitus Reaction Questionnaire). The same results were found for ongoing anxiety disorder. Whilst these figures are lower than in previous studies they are still high in absolute terms, and the lifetime prevalence for any psychiatric disturbance was 59%. This is, however, not markedly higher than what Kessler et al. (1994) found in a large community-based study of lifetime prevalence of psychiatric conditions in the general population, where almost 50% of their 8098 participants had at least one psychiatric disturbance in their lifetime.

Some studies have suggested a link between problematic tinnitus and scores on depression scales (Wilson et al., 1991), whereas others have highlighted the importance of anxiety (McKenna et al., 1996; McKenna and Hallam, 1999). Erlandsson (1990) theorized that there were two types of psychological reactions to tinnitus: one characterized by anxiety and one by depression, but these thoughts have not yet been validated empirically. As with hearing impairment, psychoacoustic measures (e.g. matching of tinnitus loudness) have not been found to be good predictors of distress (Hinchcliffe and King, 1992). Clinical experience suggests that tinnitus distress is associated with autonomic arousal, either in the form of anxiety or agitated depression, and possibly anger. Which emotion is dominant will depend on what types of beliefs the individual holds about the tinnitus. If the focus of the beliefs is about something that has been lost then depression is likely to be dominant. If it is about the possibility of future threat, or loss, then anxiety is likely to prevail. If the focus is about basic rules or assumptions being broken (e.g. 'it's not fair') then anger is likely to be uppermost.

Suicide and tinnitus

There is a popular idea that tinnitus acts as a trigger for suicide. Periodically, reports appear in the media of people with tinnitus committing suicide, and some tinnitus patients have second- or third-hand accounts of tinnitus-related suicides. There is, however, very little published scientific literature on this subject. Initial observations suggested that the incidence of suicide among patients attending a tinnitus clinic was high (Lewis et al., 1992). In a subsequent study, however, it was found that only 1.6% of people who attempted suicide had tinnitus (Lewis and Stephens, 1996), suggesting that the prevalence of tinnitus among that group of people was much less than among the general population (Axelsson and Ringdahl, 1989; Davis, 1995). None of the tinnitus cases identified in that study stated that tinnitus had played a role in their attempted suicide. These studies involved very small numbers and have several caveats associated with them, and, as a result, it is difficult to arrive at firm conclusions on the basis of their observations. Considered together, however, they do not lend strong support to the idea that tinnitus is associated with a high risk of suicide.

The characteristics of people with tinnitus who commit suicide have been reported in a small number of studies. It was reported by Lewis et al. (1992) that left-sided tinnitus was overly represented in their case series. In a later study, Lewis et al. (1994) obtained information from clinics around the world on a total of 28 people with tinnitus who had committed suicide in the preceding year. No particular tinnitus parameter, or associated audiological symptom, was overly represented in their suicide series. Stronger associations have been noted between psychological and demographic factors and suicide. People with tinnitus who commit suicide have the same sort of psychological profiles as the wider population of suicide victims (Lewis et al., 1992; Lewis et al., 1994; Frankenburg and Hegarty, 1994; Johnston and Walker, 1996). The profile is one of a history of psychiatric problems, poor current psychiatric state, being male, elderly, socially isolated, with poor social support and living in an urban environment. It might be argued that the cases described were at high risk of suicide anyway and that tinnitus is not particularly important in a suicide context. Indeed, having reviewed the literature, Jacobson and McCaslin (2001: 495) state: 'it is not tinnitus *per se* that results in suicide but concomitant psychiatric conditions that amplify the effects of tinnitus on the individual patient'. The literature does not provide evidence for a direct relationship between tinnitus and suicide, and because suicide must be mediated by psychological processes there is no basis for thinking that such a relationship might exist. In a discussion of the topic, Jacobson and McCaslin (2001) went on to assert that tinnitus does not increase the risk of suicide in depressed patients. This seems a rather sweeping assertion. It is worth noting that Lewis et al. (1994) reported that 40% of their cases had killed themselves within one year of the onset of tinnitus and approximately half had done so within two years. The expression of suicidal ideas is not uncommon among patients attending tinnitus clinics, although these are usually passive thoughts. It is also worth remembering that the psychological factors thought to be paramount in suicide, such as hopelessness, depression and anger, are often complained of by patients attending tinnitus clinics. It seems reasonable to contend that if tinnitus feeds into these psychological processes then it will add to the risk of suicide. It can be concluded that for most people tinnitus does not significantly increase the risk of suicide, but that among vulnerable patients, tinnitus (in particular of recent onset) can act as an additional stressor, in the same way as, say, unemployment, thereby increasing the risk of suicide. Professionals involved in the care of tinnitus patients should be alert to the expression of suicidal ideas in their patients. They should not be shy of enquiring further about suicidal ideas if necessary; an enquiry will not put suicidal ideas into a patient's head. If suicidal ideas are encountered, the tinnitus professional should seek immediate expert guidance, preferably from a psychologist or psychiatrist, on the management of the patient. None of this should alarm the tinnitus professional; it should be remembered that the vast majority of people with tinnitus do not suffer from significant psychological problems, let alone are not at risk for suicidal behaviour, in spite of the high prevalence of depression in clinical tinnitus patients.

Sleep

Arguably, sleep disturbance is the single most important aspect of tinnitus complaint. Evidence of the importance of sleep disturbance comes from a number of sources (McKenna, 2000). Open-ended questionnaire studies of tinnitus complaint indicate that sleep disturbance is the most common, or second most common, problem complained of (Tyler and Baker, 1983; Sanchez and Stephens, 1997). As many as 71% of tinnitus patients report sleep problems (Andersson et al., 1999). In a survey of tinnitus sufferers in New Zealand, George and Kemp (1991) found that all of their subjects indicated that tinnitus affected their sleep. On the basis of the UK National Study of Hearing, Davis (1995) reported that 5% of the population describe tinnitus that disturbs their sleep. Sleep problems are also very prevalent among children complaining of tinnitus (Gabriels, 1995). In a study of children's experiences of tinnitus, Kentish et al. (2000) reported that 80% of children referred for help with tinnitus complained of sleep problems; these problems usually being the reason that led parents to request help for their child. In an epidemiological study (n = 10 216) on sleep problems in older adults with tinnitus, it was found that poor sleep was reported by 14.4% of the men and by 27.9% of the women with tinnitus (Asplund, 2003). Interestingly, in a study on patients seen at a sleep laboratory unit, only 10 of 1500 patients had reported tinnitus, and of those only two were annoyed (Alster et al., 1993).

In addition to being very common, there is evidence that troubled sleep is the most significant complaint among tinnitus sufferers. Sleep disturbance was the largest single factor in the factor analysis of tinnitus complaint undertaken by Hallam et al. (1988), and Jakes et al. (1985) reported that difficulty sleeping was the main complaint in 50% of severe tinnitus sufferers. There is also evidence that sleep problems are associated with more distressing tinnitus. Scott et al. (1990) reported that the most important predictors of greater tinnitus discomfort and decreased tolerance of the symptom were depression and insomnia. Other researchers have reported that sleep problems are associated with more annoying and more severe tinnitus (Axelsson and Ringdahl, 1989; Hallam, 1996b; Dineen et al., 1997a; Folmer and Griest, 2000), although the relationship seemed to be a complex one.

In spite of the importance of insomnia in tinnitus complaint, it has received relatively little attention in the tinnitus research literature. It is usually referred to as just one of a number of aspects of tinnitus complaint, or outcome factors, and it has not been clearly defined in most cases. Therefore, little is known about the exact nature of the relationship between tinnitus and insomnia. Although many tinnitus sufferers believe that tinnitus prevents them from sleeping, or wakes them up in the night, it seems unlikely that tinnitus is actually a specific sleep antagonist. It is not a universal aspect of tinnitus complaint. Indeed, anecdotal clinical reports suggest that many tinnitus sufferers sleep very well. Clinical reports also suggest that the pattern of awakenings among tinnitus sufferers complaining of insomnia corresponds with the usual awakenings that are part of a normal night's sleep. These observations point to the influence of some mediating factors. It has been suggested by McKenna and Daniel (in press) that a cognitive behavioural model of insomnia can be applied in the tinnitus context and that it is anxiety associated with tinnitus, rather than tinnitus *per se*, that leads to insomnia. The ensuing anxiety about poor sleep adds to the problem, and a vicious cycle of anxiety, tinnitus and poor sleep is established in most cases. They suggested that the pre-sleep period (at the start or in the middle of the night), with its few other distractions and low levels of ambient noise, offers an opportunity to focus on tinnitus. This leads to unhelpful thoughts about tinnitus and to changes in behaviour, such as delaying going to bed when tinnitus is more intrusive, drinking alcohol and checking their tinnitus, which in turn leads to increased arousal and distress. This anxiety leads to poor sleep that, in turn, leads to further anxiety so maintaining the insomnia and the awareness of tinnitus. Whilst McKenna and Daniel (in press) emphasize anxiety as a key factor in this process these authors recognize that the anxiety may be an aspect of depression in many cases. They suggest a cognitive behavioural treatment approach.

Tinnitus and cognitive functioning

Many tinnitus sufferers complain of difficulties in cognitive functioning, in particular poor attention and concentration (Tyler and Baker, 1983; Sanchez and Stephens, 1997). As with sleep problems, there is some evidence that these difficulties are associated with more complex tinnitus involving several sounds (Hallberg and Erlandsson, 1993). Traditionally these concentration problems have traditionally been assumed to be an aspect of the emotional distress associated with tinnitus. The factor analytic studies of tinnitus complaint (Hiller and Goebel, 1992a; Hallam 1996a) did not reveal a specific 'concentration' factor, but rather suggested that cognitive difficulties form part of the emotional distress or the intrusiveness factors. This is likely to be a reflection of the fact that these questionnaires simply do not include enough questions about attention or concentration problems.

There has been a small series of studies on this hitherto neglected aspect of tinnitus complaint. The first studies (McKenna et al., 1996; McKenna, 1997; McKenna and Hallam, 1999) compared people complaining of tinnitus with people complaining of hearing loss without tinnitus on a series of clinical tests of cognitive functioning, and on a self-report measure of cognitive function, the Cognitive Failures Questionnaire (Broadbent et al., 1982). These researchers found that while the tinnitus group reported more difficulties in cognitive functioning there was only weak objective evidence of poorer cognitive performance. It appeared that the effects of tinnitus on cognitive functioning were disguised in these studies by the effects of hearing loss. Such difficulties as were apparent in cognitive functioning in the tinnitus group could not easily be explained by higher anxiety levels. In a more elaborate study Andersson et al. (2000c) compared the performance of tinnitus subjects with that of hearing-impaired control subjects, and normal subjects, on a number of Stroop tests (tests of executive functioning). Tinnitus subjects performed more poorly on all of the tests administered. The poorer performance of the tinnitus subjects could not be accounted for by differences in emotional state but, again, it was not possible to rule out some effect from hearing loss. In a recent study, Hallam et al. (2004) administered a number of computer-presented tests of cognitive function. The tests used in this study differed from those used in previous studies by these researchers in that they were experimentally based rather than tests in general clinical use. The tests assessed cognitive performance under single and dual task (carrying out the task while doing something else) conditions. In this study a group of tinnitus subjects was compared with a hearing-impaired group and also with a non-clinical control group. As in earlier studies, the tinnitus group reported more everyday cognitive failures than the control groups. The tinnitus group performed more poorly on only one objective test (the variable fore-period reaction task) under dual task conditions.

Andersson et al. (2003a) investigated autobiographical memories in 19 tinnitus patients and 19 control subjects without tinnitus. Participants were given a test of autobiographical memory, the Controlled Word Association test, and self-report measures of depression, anxiety and tinnitus distress. Compared with control subjects, tinnitus patients had difficulty retrieving specific memories and showed longer retrieval latencies. Additionally, tinnitus patients had fewer specific memories to positive cue words. This is a finding commonly observed among depressed patients (Williams et al., 1997).

The results of these studies suggest that tinnitus patients do experience some inefficiency in cognitive processing that cannot be accounted for in terms of emotional disturbance. The exact nature of the difficulties experienced is still unclear but, contrary to original expectations, it seems likely that tinnitus interferes with the performance of mundane tasks more than with high priority tasks. It is possible that tinnitus interferes with the control of attention, and in particular that it makes it more difficult to ignore things that are irrelevant to the task in hand. The work on tinnitus and cognitive function has also led to the suggestion that tinnitus can be regarded as a 'changing-state' stimulus, as it comes and goes either because of masking environmental sound or because it is a variable stimulus in itself (Andersson et al., 2002b; see also Chapter 6). This reasoning is influenced by the finding that an auditory stimulus that changes in pitch has the capacity to adversely affect cognitive processing (Jones and Macken, 1993). This view of tinnitus provides a possible explanation for patients' complaints of concentration problems, and for why some people do not manage to habituate to tinnitus.

Work

Few studies have investigated the effects of tinnitus on people's ability to work. There is the potential for tinnitus to interfere with people's ability to perform certain tasks that require precision hearing, such as the performance of classical music. As a consequence, some people with tinnitus conceal the fact that they have it. It is interesting to note that in such circumstances people often carry on working in the supposedly compromised profession. Despite the concentration problems associated with tinnitus, in practice few people are unable to work because of tinnitus itself (Andersson, 2000c). Indeed, Vallianatou et al. (2001) noted that the patients in their study group did not report that tinnitus had a detrimental effect on their ability to work. Most of their patients, however, had tinnitus of long duration and were reasonably well adjusted to it. It is also noteworthy that some people with tinnitus who are in high-profile jobs still manage to perform their duties with no apparent difficulty. In spite of these observations, some people who suffer with tinnitus do have difficulty carrying on their everyday lives, including their jobs. It seems most likely that the difficulties that such people experience can be attributed to the psychological problems associated with tinnitus (i.e. anxiety and depression) rather than the tinnitus itself.

Moderating factors

Despite the high prevalence of tinnitus, relatively few people report it to be a significant problem, and the majority of people who experience it do not seek professional help. There is therefore a question of why some people suffer much more than others. For the most part the answer is not to be found simply in the psychophysical parameters of tinnitus. Although it might be expected that particularly loud tinnitus or tinnitus of a certain frequency might lead to increased distress, this does not seem to be the case (House, 1981; Meikle et al., 1984; Kuk et al., 1990; Dineen et al., 1997a). The exception seems to be in people's subjective judgements of the complexity of the tinnitus sounds. People who experience more complex sounds report greater problems (Dineen et al., 1997a), but the cause and effect relationship is by no means clear. It has also been said that tinnitus that is present all the time has a greater impact on quality of life than tinnitus that is present for some of the time (Davis, 1995). One possible answer to why some people suffer more than others is that pre-existing psychological characteristics affect the way a person reacts to tinnitus. Several factors, including personality characteristics, coping style or ability, and emotional or psychiatric disturbance, have been the subject of investigation in this context. The psychological model outlined by Hallam et al. (1984) and the neurophysiological model proposed by Jastreboff (1990) suggested that problems arise because certain processes take place, such as changes in beliefs or unconscious classical conditioning (see Chapter 5). Problems may also arise, however, because differences in people's psychological and social background, may constitute risk factors.

The importance of differences within people's psychology in determining tinnitus distress is emphasized by the findings of a study by Attias et al. (1995). These workers found that people who sought help for tinnitus had more psychiatric problems, but lower levels of tinnitus, than people with tinnitus who did not seek help. These findings point to a relationship between tinnitus distress and vulnerability. It is possible that a more vulnerable person will be unable to tolerate even 'mild' tinnitus and even a very 'tough' person may suffer a lot when tinnitus is perceived as very loud. In other words, there is a diathesis–stress interaction taking place in which the diathesis is the vulnerability to distress, and tinnitus level is the stress.

This idea was investigated further by Andersson and McKenna (1998), who studied the relationship between depression and minimum masking levels for tinnitus. They found one group of patients with low depression and average minimum masking levels. Another group had high depression and low minimum masking levels, as predicted, but they also found a group of more depressed patients who had severe tinnitus as measured by minimum masking levels. They suggested that the lower minimum masking levels in depressed people implied that their problems were mediated by them focusing on internal sensations. The results are in keeping with a diathesis–stress model.

Gender

Gender differences in tinnitus have been reported in several studies. Women have been found to report more complex tinnitus sounds (Meikle and Griest, 1989). Although more complex tinnitus tends to be associated with more problems, it is less clear whether there are gender differences in how problematic tinnitus is. On the one hand, George and Kemp (1991) found that men reported more tinnitus-related problems than did women. On the other hand, Dineen et al. (1997a) found that women reported a greater reaction to tinnitus than did men. In a study with 146 tinnitus patients, using the Anxiety Sensitivity Index (Reiss et al., 1986), anxiety sensitivity correlated significantly with tinnitus distress ($r = 0.60$). Interestingly, the association was significantly stronger for female participants ($r = 0.74$ versus $r = 0.53$ for the males), who also scored higher on the anxiety sensitivity index (Andersson and Vretblad, 2000). In another study, Andersson and co-workers (2005) investigated the relationship between perfectionism and tinnitus distress. In addition, associations between perfectionism and sleep problems, and anxiety or depression were investigated. Gender-differentiated multiple regression analyses showed that anxiety and depressive states were related to tinnitus distress for both genders. However, for the males the perfectionism sub-scale Personal Standards was related to tinnitus distress, whereas in females it was the Organization sub-scale that was most predictive of tinnitus distress. Other studies have found no gender differences in problems related to tinnitus (Hallberg and Erlandsson, 1993). As the evidence is contradictory it is currently unwarrented to suggest that men and women with tinnitus should be managed differently.

Other somatic symptoms

The presence of other somatic symptoms may increase the burden that tinnitus patients have to bear. For example, George and Kemp (1991) found that people who experienced dizziness in addition to tinnitus reported more problematic tinnitus. In contrast to this, however, it was reported by Dineen et al. (1997a) that tinnitus subjects who experienced headaches, back pain, neck pain or balance problems reported their tinnitus to be no louder, no more annoying and no more difficult to cope with than subjects who did not have these symptoms. They did, however, find that subjects who suffered from jaw pain reported tinnitus as more annoying and more difficult to cope with, but not more loud. Notwithstanding the findings of Dineen et al. (1997a) it seems intuitively obvious that if a person has more than one problem he or she will have greater levels of distress. Indeed, McKenna et al. (1991) found greater psychological problems in neuro-otology patients complaining of more than one symptom. Although there may be greater overall distress, however, it is not necessarily the case that more symptoms will result in more problematic tinnitus. It is often the case that other symptoms, in particular dizziness, diminish the significance of tinnitus. Nonetheless, it would seem to make sense that co-existing symptoms should be tackled where possible as part of the management of the tinnitus patient.

Hearing impairment

In the population at large, the degree of hearing loss is one of the things that is most closely correlated with tinnitus (Davis, 1995). The possibility that hearing loss has some mediating influence on tinnitus must therefore be considered. The evidence about this is mixed, however. Some work has suggested that hearing loss predicts greater tinnitus distress, and the idea that hearing loss will affect tinnitus is a central tenet of the neurophysiological model of tinnitus (Jastreboff, 1990). Several studies have found that the characteristics of associated hearing loss are not associated with self-reported assessment of tinnitus (Newman et al., 1996; Meric et al., 1998; Zachariae et al., 2000; Vallianatou et al., 2001). Similarily, Scott and Lindberg (2000) found that anxiety, depression and reaction to stress in tinnitus patients remained high even when hearing impairment had been suitably rehabilitated. In other words, these problems are not related to hearing loss. Nonetheless, it seems sensible to try to alleviate a hearing loss through the use of hearing aids where one is present. Intuitively, it seems likely that if there is some external auditory input it will help to offset the internal tinnitus. The clinician needs to be aware, however, that this seemingly sensible approach has not always been successful (Melin et al., 1987).

Tinnitus and stress

There is a commonly held view that the onset of tinnitus is frequently associated with stress. This idea is actually a central tenet of the neurophysiological model of tinnitus. A common clinical observation is that tinnitus onset occurs after a period of psychological stress. There is research evidence to support this observation (Stouffer and Tyler, 1992; Schmidtt et al., 2000; Andersson et al., unpublished), which suggests that for a proportion of people the tinnitus and psychological problems occur together and, for some, the tinnitus precedes the psychological problems. Many tinnitus patients, however, relate the onset of tinnitus to noise exposure rather than stress (Meric et al., 1998) while others cannot relate the onset of tinnitus to any specific event (George and Kemp, 1991; Meric et al., 1998). The evidence on this point is therefore varied but it supports the idea that, for a substantial proportion of people, tinnitus either follows or coincides with a period of stress.

There is also the question of whether other stresses aggravate existing tinnitus. This idea is implicit in the habituation model of tinnitus described by Hallam and colleagues (1984). Most tinnitus sufferers acknowledge that stress does aggravate tinnitus, at least in so far as making it more difficult for them to cope with their symptoms. In addition to influencing tinnitus through heightening autonomic nervous system arousal it is likely that the demands of other stresses dilute a person's ability to cope with tinnitus. Some patients resist this idea, protesting that they would not be stressed if not for tinnitus, but this position is usually taken by people who are seeking a cure rather than a solution to their problems. There is also some research evidence supporting the view that stress acts as an aggravating factor for tinnitus. For example, in a study of tinnitus in air traffic controllers it was found that a high workload probably contributed to the problem (Vogt and Kastner, 2002). It was also noted, however, that difficult shift work patterns acted as a risk factor; it is possible that the disruption of the daily biorhythm played an important role in this respect. It is also acknowledged by most tinnitus sufferers that the stress associated with tinnitus aggravates the symptom, and that a vicious cycle of events is in operation. This stress arises because of the emotional connotations of tinnitus and because of the patterns of behaviour, or coping styles, that ensue.

Psychological state: anxiety and depression

The association between tinnitus and a poor psychological or psychiatric state is indisputable. It is possible to consider these psychological difficulties as either primary (i.e. causing the person to be particularly distressed by tinnitus) or as secondary to the tinnitus. Depression is a common secondary reaction to many illnesses and many patients argue that it is so with tinnitus. Despite tinnitus patients' reports of the pernicious nature of their tinnitus, however, it must be remembered that the characteristics of tinnitus do not easily predict the level of distress experienced and, therefore, if tinnitus is secondary the relationship is a complex one. There is some support for the idea that psychological problems have a primary role in the tinnitus process. In their study of tinnitus patients Sullivan et al. (1988) noted that those tinnitus patients who were depressed had more psychological and somatic complaints than tinnitus patients who were not depressed. Those tinnitus patients who were not depressed did not have more problems than the control group, strongly suggesting that tinnitus patients' problems were more closely related to the depression than to the tinnitus. It was suggested by Sullivan et al. (1988) that pragmatically it is not essential to settle the question of whether psychological problems are primary or secondary in the tinnitus process. It may be that the existence of the psychological problems is what is important rather than their primary or secondary nature. As argued by Scott and Lindberg (2000), it may be because tinnitus sufferers are more burdened by such problems that they are less able to adapt to their tinnitus. Those who are very distressed by tinnitus may fail to employ helpful strategies for coping with it. Although this suggestion returns the argument to the start of a 'cause and effect' loop, it seems clear that what is really important is that these psychological problems are treated and that tinnitus patients are not regarded simply as people with ear problems.

It was noted by Scott and Lindberg (2000) that tinnitus patients not only reported a poor psychological state (i.e. problems such as anxiety and depression) but also had greater long-term psychological problems (such as a more unhelpful dispositional style, anger and response to stress) when compared with people with tinnitus but not seeking help for it, and when compared when a normal control group. High levels of trait anxiety (i.e. a general disposition to anxiety rather than a reaction to a particular stress) among tinnitus sufferers were noted by Halford and Anderson (1991b) and by McKenna (1997). An association between the subjective severity of tinnitus and the degree of trait anxiety was noted by Halford and Anderson (1991b). The implication of this is that people who are generally more anxious are more likely to have more severe tinnitus. Arguably, someone who has an anxious and therefore negative outlook is less likely to be able to realize what coping strategies help, and will be less likely to be able to put such strategies into action. Anxiety, like depression, may also incline the person to pay greater attention to tinnitus and to have a more negative perspective on its effects. Looking at the issue from another point of view, Andersson (1996) found that a disposition towards optimism, as assessed by the Life Orientation Scale (Scheier and Carver, 1985), was negatively related to tinnitus complaints, or in other words, the greater the optimism the lower the tinnitus complaint.

Personality

More formal assessments of the personality of the tinnitus patient have also been undertaken. Personality is usually assessed by use of questionnaire measures, such as the Minnesota Multiphasic Personality Inventory (Hathaway and McKinley, 1940) or the Eysenck Personality Questionnaire (Eysenck and Eysenck, 1975). Most studies that have used such questionnaires have found that, as a group, tinnitus patients have normal personality profiles (Reich and Johnson, 1984; Collet et al., 1990; Meric et al., 1998; Vallianatou et al., 2001). Some studies have reported abnormal personality profiles in a sub-set of tinnitus patients. For example, Reich and Johnson (1984) found elevated Minnesota Multiphasic Personality Inventory schizophrenia sub-scale scores in tinnitus subjects with normal hearing. Meric et al. (1998) reported that almost half of their tinnitus subjects had at least one Minnessota Multiphasic Personality Inventory scale score beyond the normal limits. Predominantly the abnormal scale was hysteria.

The relationship between personality scores and tinnitus severity has also been investigated. A significant correlation between the neuroticism scale of the Eysenck Personality Questionnaire and Tinnitus Handicap Inventory scores was noted by Zachariae et al. (2000). Unfortunately, these researchers did not state the actual Eysenck Personality Questionnaire scores so it is not clear whether their subjects had abnormal personality profiles or not. Correlations between scores on the Minnesota Multiphasic Personality Inventory scales and scores on the Tinnitus Handicap Questionnaire and the Tinnitus Reaction Questionnaire were also found by Meric et al. (1998). The strongest correlations were with the Minnesota Multiphasic Personality Inventory depression scale. More of their subjects with abnormal Minnesota Multiphasic Personality Inventory profiles had high scores on the Tinnitus Handicap Questionnaire and Tinnitus Reaction Questionnaire than did those with normal Minnesota Multiphasic Personality Inventory profiles. It was noted by Vallianatou et al. (2001) that there was no significant relationship between personality scores and subjective rating of tinnitus intensity. It should, however, be noted that the majority of subjects in this study cannot be regarded as representative of the most problematic of tinnitus cases.

Using psychometric tests and psychiatric diagnostic methods, Erlandsson and Persson assessed a group of tinnitus patients. In addition to the presence of significant emotional distress, 50% of a sub-group of patients were diagnosed as suffering from a personality disorder. Erlandsson (2000) puts this in context by stating that 10–13% of the general population suffers from personality disorders. Phobic personality disorder and phobic tendencies were the most common diagnosis. Borderline personality disorder was confirmed in three male patients, and obsessive compulsive disorder in one female. The majority of patients were found to have two or more disorders. Patients who were diagnosed as personality-disordered did not show a change in their distress profile at subsequent review. It was suggested that tinnitus might reinforce certain personality traits in a person who is vulnerable and at the border of health and illness.

Coping style

The relationship between individual differences in coping styles and tinnitus problems has received some research attention. An early reference to the importance of coping style in adjustment to tinnitus was made by Hallam et al. (1984) when they proposed their habituation model. These authors suggested that habituation will be hindered by high levels of arousal that result from attaching emotional significance to the tinnitus. They cited 'catastrophic thinking' in particular as a factor that interferes with adjustment to tinnitus. The relationship between perceived tinnitus severity and patterns of coping style was investigated by Hallberg et al. (1992). These researchers reported that men with severe tinnitus more often engaged in 'escape coping' (e.g. wishful thinking, taking drugs or alcohol to feel better) than did men with equal hearing status but milder tinnitus or no tinnitus. These authors assessed general strategies for coping with stress rather than specific strategies for coping with tinnitus. The relationship between specific coping strategies that people used when dealing with tinnitus and the severity of tinnitus was assessed by Budd and Pugh (1996b), who used a questionnaire and factor analysis method that revealed three tinnitus coping styles. These were labelled 'maladaptive coping', 'effective coping' and 'passive coping'.

The maladaptive coping style was characterized by catastrophic thinking about tinnitus, and by ineffective attempts to avoid it by means such as daydreaming of life without it, by praying that it would go away, and also by avoiding social situations because of it. Budd and Pugh (1996b) reported that sufferers who scored highly on the 'maladaptive coping' scale reported higher levels of tinnitus severity, and more anxiety and depression than did sufferers who had a low score on this sub-scale. The passive coping style was characterized by the use of sound to mask tinnitus, by the use of relaxation techniques to cope with stress and by consulting professionals to 'offload' about the difficulties of tinnitus. There was no indication that people who scored highly on this scale accepted tinnitus, and high scores were associated with increased tinnitus severity and emotional distress. The style labelled 'effective coping' was characterized by an acceptance of tinnitus and the use of a broad range of coping strategies, such as positive self-talk, attention switching and distraction through increased activity. Curiously, this style was not associated with less severe tinnitus and there was only a small association between it and better emotional adjustment. The authors suggest that this may be because the key feature in adaptation to tinnitus is the avoidance of maladaptive coping strategies rather than the use of so-called effective ones. They point out that tinnitus distress might provoke the use of strategies such as catastrophic thinking rather than the distress being caused by such strategies. They suggest that avoiding such unhelpful strategies may allow habituation to take place. It is noticeable, however, that several of the items that make up the effective coping sub-scale are essentially forms of distraction from tinnitus, and represent avoidance behaviour which might be expected to retard adjustment.

Locus of control

A sense of personal control has been found to be an important factor when facing tinnitus and hearing impairment. The concept of 'locus of control' refers to the tendency a person has to explain events as caused by internal (within the person's responsibility) or external (outside the person's responsibility) factors. Clearly, the sense of personal control that a person has is likely to have some bearing on his or her ability to cope. It has been suggested that locus of control is one of the most important factors for health-related behaviour (Lazarus and Folkman, 1984). Personal control has also been found to be an important predictor of tinnitus discomfort and adaptation in a study by Scott et al. (1990). A significant relationship between locus of control, tinnitus severity and emotional distress in tinnitus sufferers was also found by Budd and Pugh (1995). In a study of the psychological profile of tinnitus patients, Attias et al. (1995) found that patients who sought help for tinnitus had a greater external locus of control than those who did not seek help for tinnitus. This suggests that the treatment of tinnitus patients should be aimed at facilitating coping strategies using the concept of locus of control.

Family relationships

The influence of family relationships in the experience of tinnitus has received a small amount of research interest. People who are distressed by tinnitus display a range of behaviours that communicate their distress to other people. These behaviours can come under the control of reinforcements of one kind or another from other people, in particular the patient's spouse. Thus, conceivably, a spouse who provides attention and sympathy (i.e. responds solicitously) to a patient's tinnitus behaviour may unwittingly reinforce and maintain it. Alternatively, it is possible that a spouse who ignores or punishes the tinnitus behaviour may have the effect of reducing the behaviour and so improving the patient's overall level of functioning. This process was investigated by Sullivan et al. (1994), who examined coping, depression and marital support as correlates of tinnitus disability, where disability was defined as interference with activity at work, at home and in the patient's social life. Contrary to the prediction of a conditioning model, these researchers found that punitive responses from the spouse did not have a helpful effect on the patient. They concluded that, for tinnitus patients, criticism results in demoralization rather than activation. This was particularly true when the patient experienced greater levels of depression, and Sullivan et al. (1994) suggested that in such circumstances criticism may lead to poor habituation to tinnitus. They also reported that poor marital cohesion was associated with greater disability. This study, however, focused on only one aspect of disability, namely the ability to function in very specific areas of life. Further work was done by Pugh et al. (2004), who investigated the effect of spouses' responses to patients' 'tinnitus behaviour' on the perceived severity of tinnitus, and on the level of emotional distress experienced. These workers concluded that solicitous responses on the part of spouses had a detrimental effect on the experience of chronic tinnitus, and enquiries about tinnitus tended to increase expressions of distress. They also found that punishing responses by spouses were correlated with maladaptive coping and tinnitus severity. It seems that rather than reducing tinnitus behaviours, punitive responses from spouses amounted to a removal of social support. The relationship between punitive responses and tinnitus severity appeared to be mediated by emotional distress. Interestingly, however, Pugh et al. (2004) noted that there was a direct relationship between solicitous responses and tinnitus severity as well as one mediated by emotional distress. This suggests that the influence of rewards and punishments needs to be built into any model of tinnitus distress. These researchers also found that dissatisfaction within the marriage was associated with greater anxiety and depression.

The role of family support was also investigated by Granqvist et al. (2001), who investigated the relationship between attachment patterns and tinnitus-related problems. Attachment theory originally focused on infants' ties to their mothers but has subsequently gone on to be applied in many other settings, including seeking to understand people's experiences of illness. There are two broad types of attachment patterns, referred to as 'secure' or 'insecure' (the latter being divided into avoidant or ambivalent). These researchers reported that avoidant attachment was linked to tinnitus-related problems, and that avoidant and ambivalent attachment was related to punitive family responses. Furthermore, avoidance predicted tinnitus-related problems over and above the effects of family support. Contrary to expectations, however, secure attachment patterns were not related to fewer tinnitus problems. Granqvist et al. (2001) speculated that people who have an avoidant attachment style, and who presumably perceive other people as unlikely to be able to support them, may use unhelpful coping strategies such as emotion-focused and avoidant strategies instead of problem-focused ones when dealing with tinnitus. An avoidant attachment style might also influence how a person relates to others and how others, in turn, relate to them, and hence might increase the likelihood of punitive responses from the family. Alternatively, it is possible that people high in insecurity do actually have less supportive family members because they choose partners who are similar to themselves.

Smoking, alcohol and caffeine

Many tinnitus sufferers believe that smoking, drinking alcohol, or excessive intake of drinks such as tea and coffee will influence their tinnitus. Many sufferers believe that these substances will worsen their tinnitus and are careful to abstain. Others take the view that a glass of wine or beer, or a cigarette, has a beneficial effect. The evidence linking tinnitus with any of these substances is at best equivocal. There is a suggestion that the incidence of hearing loss is greater in smokers than in non-smokers (Zelman, 1973), but a direct relationship between tinnitus and smoking still needs to be established. Similarly, no relationship between caffeine and tinnitus has been established. Nicotine and caffeine are, however, stimulants and, in theory, they might increase arousal and increase tinnitus detection through that mechanism. Alternatively, increased arousal may lead to greater anxiety levels and so reduce coping ability. This is, however, a theoretical point and anecdotal evidence suggests that few patients who cut out smoking and drinking coffee show dramatic improvements in their tinnitus.

The link between alcohol and tinnitus has received moderate research attention (McFadden, 1982; Kemp and George, 1992; Pugh et al., 1995; Stephens, 1999; Vallianatou et al., 2001) but the picture to emerge from studies is unclear. Most tinnitus sufferers report that modest alcohol consumption makes no difference to their tinnitus, but some report a temporary improvement while others report a temporary worsening. It was found by Stephens (1999) that a worsening of tinnitus after drinking alcohol was particularly noted by people who drank less alcohol; however, higher intake was found to worsen tinnitus in another study (Goodey, 1981). The consumption of alcohol was found to be a risk factor for tinnitus in a study of the epidemiology of hearing problems in Italy (Quaranta et al., 1996).

There are obvious general health benefits to stopping smoking and avoiding excessive alcohol intake but there is a risk that removing pleasures from life also reduces the rewards that might help to maintain a sense of well-being and therefore ability to cope with tinnitus.

Environment

It has been noted clinically that a change in environment can alleviate tinnitus distress. For example, some patients report an improvement in their overall well-being when they go on holiday. Unfortunately, many very distressed patients do not attempt to change their environment for fear that their ability to cope will be destabilized. This idea is never put to the test and such patients' distress persists perhaps partly as a consequence of this. Interestingly, Vallianatou et al. (2001) suggested that the agreeable environment of a Greek island may be responsible for the greater well-being of people with tinnitus who live there. Many distressed tinnitus patients who take their holidays in that part of the world would agree. A holiday, however, involves many changes, including a change in physical environment, change in stress levels, altered ambient noise levels (e.g. cicadas on a Greek island), increased alcohol intake, etc., and so it is difficult to know what the key elements involved are. Unfortunately, the reported benefits, or otherwise, of changing environment are entirely anecdotal.

Summary

It is clear then that tinnitus is associated with a variety of non-auditory problems, such as emotional disturbance, sleep problems and difficulties in cognitive functioning. It is helpful to be aware of the complexity of complaints about tinnitus for a number of reasons. It allows tinnitus workers to more properly appreciate the experiences and suffering of their patients. Without proper understanding, any attempt at therapy is likely to be much more difficult. Many patients also need to understand that their symptoms are a well-recognized part of the tinnitus experience. This appreciation is also important in a medico-legal context (McCombe et al., 2001) as it allows a proper description and grading of the severity of patients' problems. The different factors within the tinnitus complaint offer different therapeutic goals. A therapeutic effort that focuses only on the presence or absence of tinnitus is likely to be demoralizing for both patient and therapist. Goals that are set in terms of, say, changes in emotion or sleep, or some other behavioural response, are likely to be more successful. It is important to realize that, although the associations between tinnitus and these problems are usually very meaningful, the links are not always clear and proportional. In some cases, especially the suggested link between tinnitus and suicide, the suggested association is very weak or ill-founded. There is, therefore, a very real value in identifying the moderating factors which lead some people to suffer more than others. A profile of vulnerability, involving personality factors, general anxiety and crucial life stress, was identified by Erlandsson (2000). These factors, together with others such as coping style, family relationships, general health and possibly environment, may all play some part in determining the overall effect that tinnitus has on a person's life. Again, awareness of these factors may help to explain the tinnitus sufferer's experiences, in both a clinical and a medico-legal context, and if resources permit, some of these moderating factors may constitute therapeutic goals, such as a change in coping style.

Chapter 10
Hyperacusis

The terminology describing disorders of loudness perception is not consistent, due in part to the small amount of rigorous work in this area (Phillips and Carr, 1998) and in part to the observation that noise sensitivity has been described in at least four separate bodies of literature: audiology, neurology, psychiatry and in research on noise sensitivity and annoyance from a public health perspective.

Definitions and related constructs

The term 'hyperacusis' was introduced to the medical literature by Perlman (1938), and it has been defined as follows: 'unusual tolerance to ordinary environmental sounds' (Vernon, 1987) and as: 'consistently exaggerated or inappropriate responses to sounds that are neither threatening nor uncomfortably loud to a typical person' (Klein et al., 1990), underscoring the abnormality of the behavioural response to sounds. Common to both definitions is that sound of low intensity can evoke this experience, and that sounds in general (i.e. everyday sounds) are problematic rather than specific sounds. The term has almost exclusively been used in the otological and audiological literature. Although some suggestions have been given about how to measure hyperacusis, there is no consensus or empirical data today as to where to draw the line for abnormal levels of loudness discomfort for everyday sounds. It is well recognized that loudness discomfort levels have high within-subject and inter-subject variability (Stephens et al., 1977), and that they are influenced by how instructions are given in the test situation (Bornstein and Musiek, 1993), making reliable measurements difficult. However, there is some evidence that self-reported hyperacusis is accompanied by lowered thresholds for discomfort (Anari et al., 1999).

The term 'loudness recruitment' (Fowler, 1936; Moore, 1998) describes an experience commonly associated with cochlear hearing loss, and outer hair cell dysfunction in particular (Phillips and Carr, 1998). Many individuals with a cochlear hearing loss experience a rate of growth of loudness level with increasing sound level that is greater than normal (Moore, 1998). This phenomenon may be distinguished from hyperacusis if the individual experiences sound of moderate intensity as uncommonly loud (recruitment) or sound of low intensity as uncomfortably loud (hyperacusis), but the two experiences are not mutually exclusive. Loudness recruitment has not been reported to vary with mood, however. This has not yet been tested in experimental research, and it is indeed very likely that the annoyance associated with loudness recruitment is linked to mood and how the symptom is perceived.

The term 'phonophobia' has also been used for the experience of noise sensitivity and is commonly used in the neurological literature (Silberstein et al., 2001). In fact, increased noise sensitivity is a common finding in migraine, with at least 50% of attacks being accompanied by phonophobia (Woodhouse and Drummond, 1993). In addition, reduced uncomfortable loudness levels have been observed during migraine attacks (Woodhouse and Drummond, 1993). The suffix *-phobia* describes the emotional impact of disordered loudness perception, but carries the implication that the dysfunction is strongly linked with fear and hence to be considered as a psychiatric symptom. In response to this, a new word *misophonia* (Jastreboff and Jastreboff, 2003) has been proposed, deriving from the Greek for 'dislike of sound'. Although this is a laudable attempt at removing the implied phobic element while retaining the emotional aspect of the experience, the word has not been widely adopted to date. One potential reason is the fact that this new term is very close in meaning to the much more widely used concept of 'noise annoyance' in epidemiological research and therefore only adds to the terminological confusion.

Another area in which the symptom of noise sensitivity is mentioned is psychiatry. For example, the startle response is one of the symptoms used in the diagnosis of post-traumatic stress syndrome (American Psychiatric Association, 1994). The way noise sensitivity is described in the psychiatric literature often makes it indistinguishable from what audiologists understand as hyperacusis. Noise sensitivity has been observed in association with depression, leading some workers to suggest that deficits in serotonin functioning may be implicated in both depression and hyperacusis (Marriage and Barnes, 1995). In fact, given the overlap between tinnitus and depression (see Chapter 8) it would not be surprising if at least a proportion of patients with hyperacusis had diagnosable depression (Carman, 1973). Supporting this theory is the clinical observation that hyperacusis sometimes disappears once psychological well-being returns to normal.

Noise, defined as unwanted sound perceived as harmful or uncomfortable, has been studied from a public health perspective, mainly with respect to its detrimental effect on psychological well-being and on health (Job, 1996). Hence, noise sensitivity and noise annoyance have been the subject of extensive research (Abel, 1990; Stansfeld, 1992; Staples, 1996). In this literature it is common to distinguish 'noise sensitivity' and 'noise annoyance', the first being seen as an intervening variable between exposure and individual annoyance responses (Stansfeld, 1992). This distinction has not been made in the literature on hyperacusis. In community surveys a co-morbidity between noise sensitivity and psychological problems has been observed (Stansfeld, 1992), and Weinstein (1980) argued that noise sensitivity may be a personality characteristic. Stansfeld et al. (1985) suggested that between 40% and 50% of highly noise-sensitive subjects had a recognizable psychiatric disorder. Research has found that noise sensitivity is related not only to neuroticism but also to sensitivity to other aspects of the environment (Stansfeld, 1992).

Axelsson and co-workers studied the problem of hyperacusis (Axelsson et al., 1995; Anari et al., 1999) in a sample of consecutive patients referred for treatment of hyperacusis and concluded that sensitivity to sounds consists of different conditions, of which hyperacusis is one example. In the differential diagnosis of hyperacusis they proposed distinctions between hyperacusis and recruitment, distortion, psychiatric problems, noise annoyance and phonophobia. Unfortunately, this suggested categorization has not resulted in further research. The group also noted a large co-morbidity of hyperacusis and tinnitus.

In reviewing the literature on noise sensitivity and annoyance Stansfeld (1992) argued that whereas sensitivity is related to noise level, annoyance is not. From this reasoning, hyperacusis would be included under the heading of noise sensitivity, representing a particularly severe form of noise sensitivity. The distinction between phonophobia and hyperacusis has also been questioned (Marriage and Barnes, 1995), but most workers believe that the term is sufficiently distinct to be retained.

Prevalence

Epidemiological data about hyperacusis have not been robustly determined, and a search revealed only one published study in the peer-reviewed literature: this is a major shortcoming. There are, however, a few additional papers published as conference proceedings. Fabijanska et al. (1999) undertook a postal questionnaire epidemiological study of tinnitus in Poland, which included an unspecified question on hyperacusis. Of the 10 349 respondents, 15.2% reported hyperacusis, comprising 12.5% of the male respondents and 17.6% of the females. Regional differences were also reported. This report is interesting, but not sufficiently specific to be robust. This verdict also pertains to another conference report by Rubinstein et al. (1996), who described findings from a random sample of 1023 females from Gothenburg, Sweden (average age 38 years). In that study the point prevalence of hyperacusis was estimated at 23%. Unfortunately, no data on response rate or any detailed definition of hyperacusis were provided. In the only published peer-reviewed study, Andersson et al. (2002a) investigated the prevalence of hyperacusis in the adult Swedish population: a specific definition of hyperacusis was included in their questionnaire (translated from Swedish):

> In our society we are surrounded by sounds of various kinds. Some of these sounds can be annoying or even unpleasant in character. We all differ in how vulnerable we are to these sounds. In this survey we study sensitivity to everyday sounds in the sense that they evoke adverse reactions. By this we mean, for example, reactions to conversation, chirping of birds, paper noises (rustle), the ringing sound at a pedestrian crossing, or the sound of a running water-tap. In other words, we ask about sounds of moderate loudness that most people experience daily without being annoyed. Our interest is thus not restricted to loud sounds such as drilling machines or low-flying aircraft.

Two methods were utilized: first an Internet study, wherein visitors to the website of a Swedish newspaper were invited to complete a web-based questionnaire; and, second, a postal population study. Of 1167 individuals who clicked on the web banner, 595 responded, yielding a response rate of 51.9%. The point prevalence of hyperacusis in this group was 9%. The postal group comprised 987 individuals, of whom 589 responded (a response rate of 59.7%), and a point prevalence of 8% was determined. Excluding participants who reported hearing impairment resulted in point prevalence rates of 7.7% and 5.9%, respectively, in the two groups.

A co-incidence of tinnitus complaint and of experiences of hyperacusis has been widely noted. There is a consensus regarding the prevalence of hyperacusis in patients attending a tinnitus clinic with a primary complaint of tinnitus, approximating 40% (Sood and Coles, 1988; Bartnik et al., 1999; Jastreboff and Jastreboff, 2000), and in some studies up to 60% (Andersson et al., 2001). In patients with a primary complaint of hyperacusis, the prevalence of tinnitus experienced has been reported as 86% (Anari et al., 1999). However, in the epidemiological study by Andersson et al. (2002a), only 21% of the Internet group and 9% of the postal group with hyperacusis responded affirmatively to the question about tinnitus. Hyperacusis has also been suggested to be a precursor for the development of tinnitus (Hazell and Sheldrake, 1992), and as tinnitus develops it may be the case that hyperacusis becomes worse. However, in a longitudinal follow-up of tinnitus patients, sensitivity to noise became more common, increasing from 38% (Andersson et al., 1999) to 85% of the respondents (Andersson et al., 2001) five years later, which suggests that tinnitus can precede hyperacusis.

Since epidemiological findings suggest that hyperacusis is a common problem in the general population, the issue of psychiatric co-morbidity merits exploration. At the moment there is a paucity of information about the extent to which psychiatric conditions overlap with hyperacusis. There are some findings in allied disciplines and, for example, it is known that sleep problems interact with noise sensitivity in a negative way (Job, 1996). It would not be surprising if this was also relevant in hyperacusis.

Measurements of hyperacusis

Several measures of noise sensitivity exist (Zimmer and Ellermeier, 1999), including Weinstein's Noise Sensitivity Scale (Weinstein, 1980), but none of these tools particularly targets hyperacusis. Recently it has become possible to quantify the handicap associated with hyperacusis, and two instruments have been developed for this purpose. Khalfa et al. (2002) reported data from a self-report hyperacusis questionnaire with 14 items, which used normative data from 201 individuals who had answered an advertisement placed for subject recruitment. Principal component factor analysis indicated a three-factor solution accounting for 48.4% of the variance, and the three factors were identified as attentional, social and emotional. Nelting et al. (2002) reported on a questionnaire with 27 items, which used normative data from 226 patients with hyperacusis. Principal component factor analysis again indicated a three-factor solution (accounting for 50.6% of the variance) identified as cognitive reactions, actional or somatic behaviour and emotional. The latter questionnaire is presently only available in German. In neither case has the instrument yet been shown to be sensitive to treatment effects. However, the existence of such instruments is a step forward in the investigation of this phenomenon.

The type of sounds that produce hyperacusis are also pertinent: using the data from Andersson et al. (2002a) on different kind of sounds, principal components analysis showed a clear two-factor solution split with Noise, Music and Mechanical sounds forming one factor, and Talk, Paper noises and Clatter forming a second separate factor.

Without any doubt, there is a need to develop better objective measures and behavioural tests of hyperacusis, as well as further validation of self-report measures. In the literature on specific phobia, it is common to conduct behavioural tests when the phobic object is approached (Öst, 1997). This is usually also done in cognitive behavioural therapy with hyperacusis patients, but the procedures have not been tested or described in any detail in the literature. Moreover, the actual emotional and cognitive effects of exposure to sounds are virtually unexplored in hyperacusis. Another issue meriting further examination is the temporal characteristics of the sounds, as research has found that sudden noises are more likely to be viewed as aversive than constant sounds (Job, 1996).

Causes and mechanisms

A review of the medical conditions in which hyperacusis has been reported as a symptom has been undertaken by Katzenell and Segal (2001), and the conditions identified are listed in Table 10.1. It should be noted, however, that of the peripheral conditions identified, several involve facial nerve dysfunction. As the facial nerve innervates the stapedial reflex, which is a mechanism for reducing the perceived intensity of impulse sound, these conditions may reduce the efficacy of that reflex and hence increase the perceived intensity of sound. This does not meet a strict definition of hyperacusis.

Table 10.1 Medical conditions in which hyperacusis has been reported as a symptom (Katznell and Segal, 2001)

Peripheral	Central
Bell's palsy	Migrane
Ramsey Hunt syndrome	Depression
Stapedectomy	Post-traumatic stress disorder
Perilymph fistula	Head injury
Lyme disease	Williams syndrome

Lyme disease is a systemic bacterial infection that targets specific body organs, and in which both peripheral and central neurological involvement has been been observed (Coyle and Schutzer, 2002). The agent responsible is the tick-borne spirochete *Borrelia burgdorferi*, and the disease is associated with particular geographical regions where the ticks and their hosts thrive and come into contact with humans. Hyperacusis has been reported as a symptom of Lyme disease, but some caution must be exercised in view of the fact that some patients also experience a facial palsy, and hence stapedial reflex dysfunction as described above. There are reports, however, of hyperacusis in Lyme disease without facial nerve dysfunction (Nields et al., 1999).

Williams syndrome is a developmental disorder of neurogenetic basis (Levitin et al., 2003) with a prevalence of one in 20 000 live births. Affected individuals with the Williams syndrome phenotype exhibit deficits in conceptual reasoning, problem solving, motor control, arithmetic and spatial cognition (Levitin et al., 2003). Hyperacusis has been associated with Williams syndrome in up to 90% of individuals (Klein et al., 1990). The mechanism of this phenomenon has been suggested as 5-HT dysfunction (Marriage and Barnes, 1995), though the high incidence of otitis media with effusion and the associated conductive hearing loss in the Williams syndrome population may also have some influence upon auditory gain.

Within the literature there are reports of hyperacusis being associated with rare conditions, such as middle cerebral artery aneurysm (Khalil et al., 2002) and migrainous infarction (Lee et al., 2003). Although hyperacusis is not commonly associated with multiple sclerosis, a case study series has been published (Weber et al., 2003). Thus whilst hyperacusis is rarely a symptom of significant or sinister pathology, it would seem prudent that an informed clinical opinion is sought in such cases.

There are several potential mechanisms of hyperacusis. These are not mutually exclusive, and this may be a reflection of the heterogeneity of the patient population. There are at least two distinct mechanisms by which auditory gain is set in humans. The first involves the motile function of outer hair cells in the Organ of Corti within the cochlea, which is involved both in increasing the amount of activity on the basilar membrane associated with low-intensity sound, and with the fine tuning of that activity. Outer hair cells are innervated by efferent fibres from the central auditory system in large part, which analyses the sound environment and influences cochlear function accordingly. Cochlear blood flow may also be important in this process: if the cochlear blood supply is compromised the highly metabolically active outer hair cells are unable to function effectively. The second mechanism is the ability to set auditory gain within the central auditory system, based upon the observations that the range of change in gain is greater than can be accounted for purely by outer hair cell activity, and that auditory gain (and specifically auditory startle) is influenced by mood state, particularly anxiety, agitation and fear. Reciprocal links between the auditory system and the reticular formation (which influences agitation and arousal) are present at brainstem level, specifically in the superior olivary nuclei (FitzGerald and Folan-Curran, 2002). In addition, a functional connection involving the amygdalae, which are involved in fear and anxiety, and higher brainstem auditory nuclei has been described, and is thought to be involved in fear conditioning (Fredrikson and Furmark, 2003).

Several additional theories exist as possible explanations of hyperacusis. The high prevalence of hyperacusis in individuals with Williams syndrome led Marriage and Barnes (1995) to consider the mechanism in that condition, and the extent to which it might be generalized to other individuals. They suggested that a disturbance of 5-hydroxytryptamine (5-HT, serotonin) may be implicated in hyperacusis, based in part upon the clinical observation that hyperacusis is commonly co-incident with conditions where 5-HT is involved, specifically migraine, depression and post-traumatic stress disorder (Katzenell and Segal, 2001; Westcott, 2002). Serotonin does appear to have a role in modulating auditory gain and the determination of significance of sound (Thompson et al., 1994; Hurley et al., 2002). It has been noted, however, that the suggestion that the serotonin disturbance involved in hyperacusis is non-specific (Phillips and Carr, 1998) and would be difficult to subject to empirical investigation.

Another potential mechanism is that of auditory efferent dysfunction. An auditory efferent system is common to all mammals, and in humans consists of both a lateral and medial efferent system. The lateral system is characterized by having its cells of origin in or around the lateral superior olives and terminating on the primary afferent dendrites beneath the inner hair cells. The function of the lateral auditory efferent system is as yet unclear. In contrast, the cell bodies giving rise to the medial system are located medially within the superior olivary complexes and terminate on the bases of outer hair cells. The function of the medial efferent system appears to include the modulation of auditory gain (Sahley et al., 1997) and the behavioural response to sound, possibly mediated through anatomical links with the reticular formation. A role for medial auditory efferent system dysfunction in both hyperacusis and tinnitus has been mooted. It has been suggested that such dysfunction might impair the ability to modulate central gain so that the auditory system might remain at high sensitivity, even in the presence of noise of moderate to high intensity when the gain would normally be reduced (Jastreboff and Hazell, 1993). The experience of hyperacusis in patients with no apparent dysfunction or involvement of the peripheral auditory apparatus is circumstantial evidence for such central hyper-excitability. Jastreboff and Hazell (1993) further speculated that such central hyper-excitability, manifesting as hyperacusis, might represent a precursive state to troublesome tinnitus, although they did not substantiate this with data. Similar reasoning about central hyper-excitability has been undertaken in the field of chronic pain (Peters et al., 2000). There is evidence against this hypothesis, however, in that patients who have undergone vestibular nerve section (usually for symptoms of vertigo refractory to other treatments) do not complain of increased tinnitus nor loudness intolerance (Baguley et al., 2002) and, indeed, psychoacoustic testing of such patients has failed to identify any decrement in auditory performance (Scharf and Chay, 1997).

Sahley and Nodar (2001) considered the observation that hyperacusis (and tinnitus) appear to increase in extent when a person is tired, anxious or stressed. This led to the consideration of changes in the biochemical status of the cochlea, and specifically of the role of endogenous dynorphins. Sahley and Nodar (2001) proposed that during stress endogenous dynorphins might be released into the synaptic region beneath inner hair cells. This might potentiate the neurotransmitter glutamate, with the results that sound might be perceived as louder than is in fact the case – this applying both to externally generated and internally generated (tinnitus) sound. This model draws both upon biochemical knowledge about the cochlea and upon the observation that hyperacusis (and tinnitus) are exacerbated by stress, but empirical evidence in support of this theory has not yet been forthcoming.

A psychological model for hyperacusis uses the concept of classical conditioning of emotional responses to sound (Schwartz, 1989). Sounds can become associated with aversive responses involving the limbic and autonomous nervous systems, although the auditory system is functioning normally (Jastreboff, 2000). This 'fear of sound' is commonly seen among patients with hyperacusis, and the aversive reactions may occur in response to certain sounds whereas other sounds of similar levels are not feared. However, the idea that hyperacusis may involve fear of injury to the auditory system has not been explored. In the literature on chronic pain, the fear-avoidance model (Lethem et al., 1983; Vlaeyen and Linton, 2000) has become well established. This model predicts that the fear of pain may serve a causal role in leading to disability in that fear of injury leads to inactivity and that inactivity in itself leads to even more pain and disability. The parallel in hyperacusis is that avoidance of auditory stimulation is likely to sensitize the auditory system which, in turn, exacerbates the hyperacusis. Hence, as gradual exposure to feared movements have been endorsed in pain management programmes (Vlaeyen et al., 2001), gradual exposure to sound has been recommended in the treatment of hyperacusis (Vernon, 1987b; Jastreboff, 2000; Sammeth et al., 2000). A comprehensive model for understanding hyperacusis should involve consideration of sensitivity, annoyance and fear of injury. The first two have been extensively researched in the literature on noise sensitivity (Stansfeld, 1992), and fear of injury could be a distinguishing factor in hyperacusis. Following this reasoning, hyperacusis can be seen from three different angles, depicted in Figure 10.1. In this model, the experience of hyperacusis can involve annoyance and irritation, without necessarily having a sense of being harmed (e.g. irritation caused by neighbours playing music). It can also involve somatic sensations of pain and otalgia, when sounds are experienced as pain in the ear. Lastly, hyperacusis may involve a sense of hearing being harmed or, in the case of concurrent tinnitus, that tinnitus might become worse. The fear may concern specific sounds, or sound in general. The links between the central auditory system and areas of the brain implicated with anxiety and fear are currently being investigated. Specifically, anatomical and functional links between the central auditory system and the amygdalae have been identified (Bhatnagar, 2002), this being an essential element of fear conditioning.

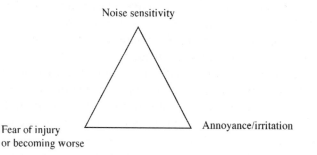

Figure 10.1 A three-component model of hyperacusis.

Treatment

For many patients, the first reaction to hyperacusis is to use earplugs, ear muffs or other hearing protection devices in order to protect them. As most of the theories of hyperacusis suggest that it is a disorder of central gain, the use of such devices, which decrease the intensity of sound entering the auditory system, may actually increase central gain further, and thus exacerbate the problem rather than improve it.

Clinicians have frequently failed to recognize hyperacusis as a genuine symptom, and seem unaware of therapeutic options. This is understandable given the dearth of published research about hyperacusis, and the complete absence of randomized controlled trials on the subject. However, there are some management strategies, and preliminary findings are promising. The most commonly used techniques are tinnitus retraining therapy and cognitive behavioural therapy, but pharmacologically based treatments might be helpful in selected cases associated with specific pathology, such as Lyme disease.

Tinnitus retraining therapy has been advocated as a treatment for hyperacusis as well as tinnitus (see Chapter 12). Following audiological and medical evaluation, the treatment protocol (Jastreboff and Jastreboff, 2000) requires classification of the patients according to their hyperacusis state, and then 'directive counselling' about the auditory system and understandings of mechanisms of hyperacusis and the associated distress. Sound therapy in the form of binaural ear level wide-band sound generators is undertaken, even when the symptoms are unilateral. The mechanism by which this sound therapy might be effective is said to be desensitization, and the sound intensity is increased from a low level very gradually over time. Retraining therapy for hyperacusis has not yet been subject to randomized placebo-controlled trials, but Sammeth et al. (2000) found some evidence of its effectiveness in a few cases. In addition, several observational studies (Gold et al., 2002, Hazell et al., 2002) indicate improvements in loudness tolerance, but these have not been published in peer-reviewed journals.

The approach taken by tinnitus retraining therapy practitioners, of encouraging the understanding and insight of patients about their situation, and the use of low-level, non-threatening, wide-band noise seems based on common sense. Unfortunately, because the natural history of hyperacusis is poorly understood, placebo effects cannot be excluded. Although most reports of the use of tinnitus retraining therapy in the management of hyperacusis are positive, there is one report by Axelsson et al. (1995) that is less encouraging. Despite this, the tinnitus retraining therapy approach is promising.

Hyperacusis has also been treated using cognitive behavioural therapy, which can be used to treat the emotional, anxiety and stress issues involved in hyperacusis. Advice regarding hyperacusis is included as a standard component in the cognitive behavioural therapy treatment of tinnitus provided at Uppsala University, but there is a shortage of studies specifically targeting hyperacusis in isolation. However, Scott (1993) reported beneficial results in a conference case report involving gradual exposure. Gradual exposure to sound has been recommended for hyperacusis, and a few case studies have been reported showing beneficial results (Vernon, 1987a; Gabriels, 1993).

There is a certain amount of controversy between the respective advocates of tinnitus retraining therapy and cognitive behavioural therapy.

However, in the management of hyperacusis the differences between the two techniques are not marked, and elements of both approaches may be appropriate.

Summary

Whilst this area has previously been under-researched there has been considerable progress evident in recent years. Terminology is becoming better defined, and hypotheses about mechanisms of hyperacusis are becoming better constructed and congruent with modern neurophysiological and biochemical insights. Treatment strategies are available, and evidence regarding their efficacy is emergent. Although there are very significant gaps in knowledge about hyperacusis, this review of current perspectives gives hope for increased understanding and treatment efficacy. However, further progress necessitates that different communities communicate better; hypercusis is a typical example of an area in which researchers and clinicians have failed to communicate across their interdisciplinary boundaries.

Chapter 11
Traditional treatments

Many therapeutic options have been considered in the management of tinnitus, including surgical treatments, drug treatments, psychological techniques and physical therapies, and many of them are still practised, though often their evidence base is weak or completely lacking. In this chapter some of the more commonly used modalities are considered. Therapies that fall outside the umbrella of conventional medicine are discussed in Chapter 14, which focuses on the use of complementary medicine in tinnitus management.

Surgical treatment

Surgery has a definite role to play in those patients whose tinnitus arises as part of syndromes such as Ménière's disease, otosclerosis and vestibular schwannoma. This is discussed in Chapter 4, as is the surgical management of objective tinnitus. Only surgery for non-syndromic tinnitus is considered here. There are two main types of surgery that have been tried for non-syndromic tinnitus: destructive procedures on the auditory system and operations that decompress the auditory nerves.

Destructive operations

Attempts to cure tinnitus surgically by creating lesions within the auditory system have generally concentrated on the cochlea and the cochlear nerve, although in 1965 Beard investigated the effects of leucotomy on tinnitus. Surgical management of tinnitus by nerve section has been reported, with either division of the whole VIIIth nerve or selective division of the cochlear nerve, sparing the vestibular nerves (Wazen et al., 1997). By retaining the vestibular nerves the incidence of post-operative nausea, vomiting and vertigo is reduced.

The results of cochlear neurectomy are variable and generally improve the tinnitus in about half of the patients. Pulec (1995) reported a series of 151 patients who had undergone cochlear neurectomy for tinnitus: total resolution or partial improvement of the tinnitus was reported in 95% of the patients, but unfortunately the results were not based on established outcome measures. There is an international consensus that cochlear neurectomy should be considered only for those patients who have no useful remaining hearing in the affected ear and who have exhausted absolutely all non-operative treatment options. If the patient has bilateral complete hearing loss, cochlear implantation is undoubtedly a better option as it offers the chance of both improved communication and reduced tinnitus.

Decompressive operations

Compression of cranial nerves by adjacent blood vessels has been suggested as a cause of several conditions, including trigeminal neuralgia, hemifacial spasm and certain forms of tinnitus (Møller, 1998). The pressure of the vessel is thought to damage the nerve, leading to secondary changes within the central auditory pathways (Schwaber and Whetsell, 1992). Specific operative techniques have been developed for microvascular decompression of the VIIIth nerve in the cerebellopontive angle (Brookes, 1996; Jannetta, 1998). Improvement of tinnitus post-operatively varies from 40% (Brookes, 1996) to 77% (Møller et al., 1993).

As most patients with non-syndromic tinnitus have neither a profound sensorineural hearing loss nor vascular compression of the VIIIth cranial nerve, the role of surgery is extremely limited.

Pharmacological

Research into drug treatment of tinnitus should be relatively easy to undertake, as it is much easier to perform randomization and to select suitable control subjects for drug therapy than for treatments such as surgery, psychological therapies or tinnitus retraining therapy. However, there are many different pathophysiological processes which can result in tinnitus, and individual patients with tinnitus can have very different experiences of the symptom. Tinnitus patients are likely to present very heterogeneous characteristics in a similar way to chronic pain patients (Møller, 1997). This heterogeneity bedevils research into drug treatment of tinnitus. Many large studies of both conventional and complementary drug therapies fail to show statistical benefit to the treatment group. However, it is possible that small sub-groups of patients with specific aetiological factors are deriving benefit but the effect is being lost within the larger population. Numerous pharmacological agents have been assessed for potentially beneficial action in tinnitus patients (Murai et al., 1992; Simpson and Davies, 1999) but relatively few have received the rigorous scrutiny of a randomized control trial (Dobie, 1999).

Local anaesthetics

One of the tantalizing success stories of tinnitus treatment is the positive response of many patients to an intravenous bolus injection of local anaesthetic agents such as lidocaine (previously known as lignocaine in some countries). This effect was first recognized serendipitously by Bárány (1935) when procaine, being used as a local anaesthetic in a nasal operation, caused tinnitus relief in the patient. The effect was investigated by Lewy (1937) and subsequent work has confirmed the phenomenon (den Hartig et al., 1993).

Lidocaine ameliorates tinnitus for a limited period of time in approximately 60% of sufferers (Simpson and Davies, 1999). The chief therapeutic application of lidocaine is as a local anaesthetic agent, in which case it is given topically or regionally. It is also useful, given intravenously, in the treatment of some cardiac dysrhythmias. In these circumstances lidocaine has a membrane-stabilizing action due to antagonism of sodium channels. This mechanism may not apply to its effect in tinnitus and it has been suggested that the action on tinnitus is mediated by altering serotonin (5-hydroxytryptamine or 5-HT) function (Simpson et al., 1999). When used in the experimental treatment of tinnitus, lidocaine is generally given at a dosage of 1 mg/kg of body weight, as a slow intravenous injection over a period of several minutes. Any tinnitus-suppressing effect is usually brief because of the short half-life of the drug within the circulation. There are also potentially serious side effects of administering the drug intravenously, with convulsions, respiratory depression, hypotension, bradycardia and cardiac arrest listed as possible. In addition, lidocaine is not licensed for the treatment of tinnitus in most countries. For these reasons, lidocaine is not suitable for general tinnitus management. The effect of other local anaesthetic agents with similar modes of action, such as procaine (Fowler, 1953) and bupivicaine (Weinmeister, 2000) have been reported but these have similar drawbacks. There are some sodium channel antagonists that can be administered orally, and there was initial hope that these would prove efficacious in the management of tinnitus; for example, tocainide (Blayney et al., 1985) was tried to no avail. Similarly, intra-tympanic injections of lidocaine proved ineffective (Coles et al., 1992) and in any case were too unpleasant to justify as a regular therapeutic option.

Psychoactive drugs

The psychoactive drugs include compounds which act on receptors that are common within the central auditory pathways. Therefore some of these drugs might be expected to be active against tinnitus. However, both depression and anxiety are commonly seen in tinnitus patients and it is frequently impossible to decide if the mood change has followed the tinnitus or vice versa. It is similarly very difficult, when conducting trials on psychoactive drugs, to ascertain whether the drug is affecting the tinnitus directly or is affecting the mood disturbance, and is thereby having a secondary beneficial effect on the tinnitus. Consequently, there are conflicting reports of the efficacy of psychoactive drugs in the management of tinnitus.

Tricyclic antidepressants

In the first published trial of the use of tricyclic antidepressants in the treatment of tinnitus Mihail et al. (1988) found no clear effects when using trimipramine. Sullivan et al. (1993) reported positive effects in a study involving 92 tinnitus patients who were given either nortriptyline or placebo. Interestingly, some reductions in loudness were observed. Also of interest was the size of the placebo effect in this trial: 40% of the group receiving the placebo reported benefit. If tinnitus patients have associated depression and insomnia, amitriptyline remains useful as it has quite marked sedating effects. A trial by Bayar et al. (2001) showed amitriptyline to be beneficial in the overall management of tinnitus but no attempt was made to separate the depressive symptoms from the tinnitus complaint. Overall, it seems likely that tricyclic drugs alleviate the distress of tinnitus rather than having any specific effect on the condition.

Selective serotonin reuptake inhibitors

Serotonin is a common neurotransmitter in the central auditory system and has a suggested role in the pathogenesis of some forms of tinnitus (see Chapter 7). Therefore, drugs that modulate serotonin activity might be expected to influence tinnitus. A recent study by Folmer et al. (2002) found that 33.8% of 957 patients attending a tinnitus clinic reported that they had depression at the time of referral to the clinic. At this time, 11.0% of the patients were taking selective serotonin reuptake inhibitor medication. Thirty patients who had started the selective serotonin reuptake inhibitors after the onset of the tinnitus were examined in more detail and it was discovered that both the depression and tinnitus improved while they were on the selective serotonin reuptake inhibitors. However, the patients also received psychotherapy during this period so it is not possible to ascribe all the benefit to the drugs.

Benzodiazepines

Benzodiazepines, such as diazepam, lorazepam and alprazolam, are drugs with sedating and hypnotic properties. They bind to receptors associated with receptors for the inhibitory neurotransmitter gamma aminobutyric acid (GABA) and have been used extensively in the management of tinnitus. A well constructed trial by Johnson et al. (1993) attempted to separate direct tinnitus suppression from the generalized anxiolitic actions of alprazolam, and demonstrated tinnitus reduction in 76% of the trial patients. Szczepaniak and Møller (1996) suggested that benzodiazepines might suppress tinnitus by reducing neural overactivity in the inferior colliculus. Unfortunately, benzodiazepines have proved to induce both physical and psychological dependence, limiting their usage.

Antispasmodic agents

Baclofen is a GABA agonist that has antispasmodic properties. Because the mechanism of action has similarities to the action of the benzodiazepines it was hoped that it would be effective in tinnitus control but be free of addictive side effects. Unfortunately, trials have shown it to be ineffective in tinnitus management (Westerberg et al., 1996).

Anti-epileptic agents

Anticonvulsant medications act by reducing hyper-excitability within the central nervous system and because of this it was hoped that they would also prove active against hyper-excitability within the auditory system. Carbamazepine is a sodium channel blocker, in many ways similar to the local anaesthetic drugs, and active when taken orally. Unfortunately, a study by Donaldson (1981) showed little useful effect in tinnitus. However, Sanchez et al. (1999) have suggested that if patients are selected on the basis of a positive response to a trial dose of intravenous lidocaine they are then likely to respond favourably to carbamazepine. Other anticonvulsant agents, including amino-oxyacetic acid (Reed et al., 1985), caroverine (Denk et al., 1997) and lamotrigine (Simpson et al., 1999) have been assessed for tinnitus-supressing activity. Caroverine showed some therapeutic effect but had to be administered by intravenous infusion.

Vasodilators

The rationale for the use of vasodilators in the treatment of tinnitus is that increasing the perfusion of the cochlea and brain should enhance the supply of oxygen and nutrients, and reduce any dysfunction. The cochlea derives its arterial supply from the inferior cerebellar artery, which is part of the cerebral circulation. The cerebral circulation possesses a robust autoregulation mechanism that keeps perfusion within quite tight parameters, irrespective of the state of the peripheral circulation. Therefore it is unlikely that many vasodilators can have significant effect on cochlear function. Nimodipine is a calcium L channel-blocking drug that does possess activity for cerebral blood vessels. One study (Theopold, 1985) suggested that it was effective in tinnitus management but a later study (Davies et al., 1994) failed to replicate these findings. Betahistine is a histamine analogue that has been promoted for the treatment of Ménière's disease and is thought to improve cochlear blood flow. There is no evidence for any beneficial effect among patients with other forms of tinnitus. Despite this it is frequently dispensed by primary care physicians for non-syndromic tinnitus and at least has the benefit of being reasonably free of serious side effects.

Diuretics

Diuretics, such as furosemide (previously known as frusemide in some countries) (Jayarajan and Coles, 1993), and osmotic diuretics, such as mannitol and glycerol (Filipo et al., 1997), have been studied but do not seem to have major benefit in the treatment of tinnitus.

Treatment by masking

Tinnitus masking involves the use of wearable ear-level devices that deliver sound to the patient's ears. The purpose is to produce a sense of relief by making the tinnitus inaudible or by changing its characteristics. Masking has been one of the most commonly applied means of dealing with tinnitus (Vernon and Meikle, 2000) and was suggested as early as 1928 (Jones and Knudsen). As discussed in Chapter 6, total masking of tinnitus is at best tedious and sometimes impossible. Sound therapy is used at much lower levels in tinnitus retraining therapy, in which case it is referred to as 'sound enrichment', and to help to distinguish between masking and the tinnitus retraining therapy approach, exponents of tinnitus retraining therapy use the term 'sound generator' instead of 'masker'. The use of sound therapy in tinnitus retraining therapy is discussed in Chapter 12. In this section classical masking is discussed, together with the effects of masking by means of hearing aids.

Masking devices and their effects on tinnitus have been studied extensively (Vernon, 1977) and much research questions their efficacy. In an ambitious multicentre study (Hazell et al., 1985) few positive effects were found, and even fewer were found in a controlled study embedded within that study (Stephens and Corcoran, 1985). In another controlled study, with placebo maskers, Erlandsson et al. (1987) found no differences between masking and placebo. Lastly, masking has not been found to boost the benefits of psychological treatment (Jakes et al., 1992). As another caveat, it has been observed that many patients (up to 50%) do not accept masking as a treatment (Vernon et al., 1990; Henry et al., 2002a). In theory, total masking is said to prevent habituation (Jastreboff and Jastreboff, 2003). There is little if any experimental research on tinnitus patients to support this hypothesis, although it remains plausible. Studying masker treatment is hindered by the observation that masking was rarely practised in isolation and patients receiving maskers often received other treatment modalities, such as counselling (Henry et al., 2002a).

The possible benefit of using hearing aids to obtain relief from tinnitus was commented on in 1947 by Saltzman and Ersner. Initial uncontrolled studies suggested that tinnitus patients were helped by hearing aids (Stacey, 1980; Surr et al., 1985), but in a later controlled study no positive effects were found (Melin et al., 1987). In a more recent uncontrolled study by Surr et al. (1999), hearing aid use was found to be associated with reduced tinnitus handicap, but the authors admitted that the effect was small. The effect of digital hearing aids upon tinnitus is of interest and warrants careful investigation.

There are also combination instruments, in which a hearing aid and a masker are housed in the same unit. There is a dearth of good experimental evidence about their efficacy and they are notoriously difficult to fit and maintain.

Electrical stimulation and cochlear implants

Electrical stimulation of the ear, especially when direct current stimulation is used, can reduce or abolish tinnitus (Dauman, 2000). However, it has proved problematical trying to turn this experimental observation into a clinically useful tool as it is difficult to get sufficient electrical power to the inner ear without causing damage. External electrical stimulation has proved beneficial in the treatment of chronic pain and has given rise to the clinically useful technique of transdermic electrical nerve stimulation (TENS). Similar techniques have been assessed in tinnitus patients (Chouard et al., 1981; Schulman, 1985; Lyttkens et al., 1986). In a placebo-controlled trial by Dobie et al. (1986) 20 patients were given either proper stimulation or placebo in a double blind cross-over trial. Severity of tinnitus decreased for two patients following the active treatment, but four patients in the placebo condition also reported improvement, suggesting that any positive response could be explained by the placebo effect. Interestingly, however, one patient derived marked benefit, and a prolonged study with this patient seemed to suggest that the effect was not attributable to placebo in this individual. Therefore there may be a limited role for this type of therapy. Following observations on chronic pain patients, there have been other studies in which sites distant from the ear have been stimulated in an attempt to alleviate tinnitus. Kaada et al. (1989) applied low-frequency electrical stimulation to the arms of 29 patients with tinnitus. Nine patients reported reduced tinnitus and, of these, seven had improved hearing. However, the study was inadequately controlled and it is difficult to extrapolate generally. There have been some anecdotal reports of stimulation of the deep external auditory canal supplying tinnitus relief and this area probably merits further research.

Surgical implants into the middle or inner ear are too invasive to be considered for widespread usage among tinnitus patients who have useful hearing. However, such objections do not apply to patients who have already lost all their hearing: ever since cochlear implantation became possible there has been much interest in its effect on tinnitus among patients with profound sensorineural hearing loss. Initial reports studied the effects of promontory stimulation and then single channel cochlear implantation. More recent work has looked at the effects of multichannel implants and this has been reviewed by Quaranta and colleagues (2004). Tinnitus is experienced by up to 86% of adult cochlear implant candidates, but is not universal and is only bothersome in a small proportion. Electrode insertion may induce tinnitus in a small (up to 4%) number of patients, but this is rare. Cochlear implant device usage is associated with reduction of tinnitus intensity and awareness in up to 86%, and rarely with exacerbation (up to 9%). There are some indications in the literature that the more complex the simulation strategy the larger that beneficial effect. Interestingly, unilateral cochlear implant usage is generally associated with reduction of contralateral tinnitus (in up to 67% of individuals) rather than exacerbation, which undermines the assertion (Jastreboff, 2000) that unilateral sound therapy for tinnitus is contraindicated.

It should be noted that cochlear implant stimulation strategies are designed to optimize speech perception, but they may not be optimal for tinnitus inhibition. Daumann et al. (1993) undertook some preliminary experiments with two cochlear implant subjects with tinnitus in an attempt to identify which combination of stimulation rate and location was most effective in suppression of tinnitus. Rubenstein et al. (2003) reported the efficacy of electrical stimulation with 5000 pps pulse trains via cochlear implant (three subjects) and via a transtympanic electrode (11 subjects), reporting that 'between a third and a half of them achieve clinically significant tinnitus suppression without a sustained percept'. Vernon and Meikle (2000) reported a case where masking bilateral tinnitus with noise (from 6 kHz to 14 kHz) via a Nucleus 22 cochlear implant was helpful, leading to some residual inhibition lasting two to three minutes and some reported contralateral suppression. This remains an interesting area.

Biofeedback

In some patients who find traditional relaxation therapy unhelpful, biofeedback has clinical utility. This technique allows the patient to monitor the stress level, usually measured by galvanic skin response, with either an auditory or visual signal (Young, 2000). The literature in this area is equivocal (Dobie, 1999; Andersson and Lyttkens, 1999). Biofeedback can be useful for tinnitus patients who are profoundly deaf, and who find the 'eyes closed, lying on the bed' methods of relaxation therapy troubling. Early studies using a biofeedback method in which warmth of the fingers and muscle tension in the forehead were monitored produced optimistic results (House et al., 1977; House, 1978). However, these trials were not controlled, and along with other uncontrolled studies (Carmen and Svihovec, 1984; Walsh and Gerley, 1985; Ogata et al., 1993) the positive findings reported must be interpreted with caution. Among the available controlled trials the findings are less supportive, with a trial by Haralambous et al. (1987) showing non-significant effects. A trial by Podoshin et al. (1991) showed that biofeedback techniques were more efficacious in tinnitus control than the use of acupuncture or cinnarizine. White et al. (1986) studied 22 patients who received biofeedback for their tinnitus and concluded that the results in the test group were significantly better than those in the control group. However, the test group also received relaxation therapy, which somewhat dilutes the findings.

In one interesting study by Ince et al. (1987) an auditory matching-to-sample feedback technique was used for training self-control of tinnitus. Patients were trained to decrease the volume of their tinnitus by first matching to an external sound and then decreasing the volume of that sound while trying to decrease their own tinnitus sound. It was reported that 84% managed to decrease the loudness of the tinnitus between 10 decibels and 62 decibels. Unfortunately, this study has not been replicated and it raises several concerns about measurement of loudness and residual inhibition. Still, the approach was innovative and could potentially be helpful.

In summary, biofeedback has been researched sparsely with regard to its effect on tinnitus and is sometimes overly criticized (Howard, 2001, see Baguley and Andersson, 2002).

Relaxation training therapy

Relaxation therapy has long been viewed as an important part of tinnitus management. Therapy may be delivered in groups, or by individual instruction, or administered through use of tape recordings. Reasonable evidence for the efficacy of relaxation therapy is available (Andersson and Lyttkens, 1999; Dobie, 1999). However, relaxation can be presented in many different ways, and it is therefore important to look at the evidence of how well relaxation works as sole intervention. Commonly, relaxation is presented as one out of many treatment ingredients in the psychological management of tinnitus (Chapter 13), and in particular the method of applied relaxation (Öst, 1987), which forms part of the treatment protocol in Uppsala, Sweden (Andersson, 2001). There are two controlled studies in which relaxation has been studied as an isolated treatment modality. There were only minor effects of relaxation in a study by Ireland et al. (1985), but this study was of limited statistical power (for meta-analysis of the findings, see Andersson and Lyttkens, 1999). In another small trial, Davies et al. (1995) compared cognitive therapy, passive relaxation and applied relaxation. Results showed superior outcome of cognitive therapy and applied relaxation compared with the passive relaxation but, at four-month follow-up, improvements had disappeared. Again, as previously stated, relaxation has often been included as an element of other treatment approaches (Dineen et al., 1997b), but from the literature it appears as if relaxation on its own is of marginal benefit for tinnitus patients. The results concerning applied relaxation fare better, but this is a more comprehensive treatment in which daily practice is encouraged. It is not an easy task to disentangle different approaches to relaxation, and yoga (Kröner-Herwig et al., 1995) for example, has been considered under the umbrella of relaxation therapy. Recently, beneficial effects on immune functioning were observed in a study on the effects of progressive relaxation for tinnitus patients (C. Weber et al., 2002).

Hypnotherapy

Hypnotherapy was first suggested as a therapeutic option for tinnitus by Pearson and Barnes (1950) and there has been background interest since that time (Dobie, 1999). There are striking similarities between hypnosis and some techniques used in cognitive behavioural therapy for tinnitus, but in the present context it is important to underscore the fact that hypnosis is a well established treatment technique (Kihlstrom, 1985) that is not to be mistaken for the way hypnosis is presented in showbusiness. The aim of hypnosis is to let the mind reach a more focused and relaxed state. In addition, hypnosis can alter somatic experience to the extent that pain is decreased. There are methods in which self-hypnosis is used, which for some patients is easier to grasp than is the concept of being hypnotized. There are a number of case reports on the use of hypnosis for tinnitus (Marlowe, 1973; MacLeod-Morgan et al., 1982). In a Swedish open study, Brattberg (1983) described the application of hypnosis supplemented by tape-recorded relaxation instructions. She noted that 22 of 32 patients benefited from the treatment, but no established outcome measures were used. In a crossover study, Marks et al. (1985) studied 14 patients and used three different forms of relaxation. Only five patients reported that the treatment had helped them. Interest in hypnosis has continued and Attias and co-workers in Israel conducted two studies on the effects of self-hypnosis. In the first study, these authors included 36 patients who were randomized to three groups: self-hypnosis, masking, and waiting list control (Attias et al., 1990). The treatment groups received four sessions and then the outcome was evaluated. In addition, a two-month follow-up was included. Results showed that 73% were improved and that the results were maintained at follow-up. In a replication, the same research group included 44 patients and randomized them into three groups (Attias et al., 1993b). The main difference was that they did not include a waiting list control group, but instead an attention control group, whose members had the opportunity to discuss their tinnitus in a group without any direct intervention. All participants received five weekly sessions. The self-hypnosis group also received a cassette tape and were instructed to listen to the recording of the session and to practise. Again, self-hypnosis resulted in improvements, whereas masking did not have any effect. Surprisingly, the attention control group improved on some measures. One problem with the studies by Attias et al. is that they did not utilize well-established or validated outcome measures. Other studies suggest that hypnosis should be considered in the treatment of tinnitus (Kaye et al., 1994; Mason and Rogerson, 1995; Mason et al., 1996).

Psychodynamic and supportive therapy

Although cognitive behavioural psychotherapy has dominated the psychotherapy research scene with regard to tinnitus and in many other areas (Barlow, 2001), psychodynamic approaches are spread worldwide and still represent the most commonly practised form of psychotherapy (Seligman, 1995). Psychodynamic approaches are heterogeneous, influenced to a variable extent by the writings of the founder of psychoanalysis, Sigmund Freud. In the main, therapy is targeted towards underlying conflicts and relationship issues. Concepts such as transference (patient's attitude towards the therapist) and counter-transference (how the therapist reacts towards the patient) are central for treatment. Commonly, psychodynamic treatments are less symptom-oriented (Roth and Fonagy, 1996). No psychodynamically informed treatment has been developed for tinnitus, but early case studies have been published (Weinschel, 1955; Schneer, 1956). Despite the lack of empirical support, it is likely that some aspects of psychodynamic and supportive therapies could be beneficial for tinnitus patients. For example, Granqvist et al. (2001) found a relation between attachment and tinnitus distress. Overall, interpersonal issues have not been targeted in treatment research on tinnitus, and the role of non-specific support is not clearly established.

Summary

Numerous treatments have been tried in an attempt to cure or ameliorate tinnitus. Sadly, few seem to have any beneficial effect and even those that at first glance seem to help, rarely stand up to rigorous scientific scrutiny. Surgical treatments of non-syndromic tinnitus are rarely justified, with the notable exception of cochlear implantation for profoundly deafened tinnitus sufferers. There have been tantalizingly optimistic results from drug therapy, in particular with lidocaine and some psychoactive medications. More research is needed in this area. Treatment with maskers has failed to demonstrate long-term success but does allow some patients to obtain temporary respite from their symptoms. Biofeedback and relaxation training are related methods that do offer some help but evidence that they work as stand-alone treatments is poor and they probably need to be embedded within a more comprehensive management plan. Hypnotherapy is potentially a useful tool in tinnitus management and merits further consideration. Unfortunately, there is a dearth of hypnotherapists with interest and experience in treating tinnitus. Despite the poor evidence base for genuine effectiveness of conventional treatments, the strong placebo effect in tinnitus management ensures that many people treated with these modalities do appear to derive benefit. The simple fact that a healthcare professional is trying to help, and doing so in a caring and understanding fashion, should not be underestimated.

Chapter 12
Tinnitus retraining therapy

The publication of the Jastreboff neurophysiological model (Jastreboff, 1990) represented a synthesis of knowledge about the auditory system, and of related systems of emotion and reaction, and how these are involved in the development and persistence of distressing tinnitus. Published as it was, in a neuroscience journal, it would have been read and cited by that community, but it is unlikely that it would have attracted such widespread interest, particularly from the clinical community, if it had not been for the interaction between Pawel Jastreboff and Jonathan Hazell, an English otolaryngologist who had long specialized in tinnitus. Their early discussions had resulted in a review paper (Hazell and Jastreboff, 1990) that contained information about the medical and surgical management of tinnitus, and also on the practical, clinical implications of the neurophysiological model. Further influence upon the development of a clinical protocol congruent with the Jastreboff model was provided by Jacqui Sheldrake, a UK-based audiologist who had lengthy experience in the treatment of tinnitus patients.

A detailed consideration of the practical implications of the Jastreboff model was undertaken by Jastreboff and Hazell (1993), this paper being more accessible to clinicians than the original publication (Jastreboff, 1990). Fundamental to the neurophysiological model is the concept that tinnitus is perceived because of a failure of filtering mechanisms at a subcortical level (see Chapter 5), and that the symptom becomes distressing because of the involvement of systems of emotion and reaction (the limbic system and autonomic nervous systems, respectively). The implication, therefore, is that the filtering mechanisms might be modified or retrained so that they once more become effective at filtering the tinnitus. Furthermore, the emotional and reactive components of tinnitus complaint might be reduced by influence upon the meaning of the tinnitus. Both then (Jastreboff and Hazell, 1993) and now (Jastreboff and Jastreboff, 2003) Jastreboff and Hazell have promoted the theory that the development of tinnitus-related distress involves a traditional conditioned response paradigm.

In their 1993 consideration of the clinical implications of the neurophysiological model Jastreboff and Hazell proposed intervention for distressing tinnitus with a protocol which should include:

- 'Cognitive therapy' (Jastreboff and Hazell, 1993: 13), which they also entitled 'directive counselling' to facilitate understanding of tinnitus.
- Sound therapy to promote the plasticity of brainstem filtering systems using white noise delivered by ear-level devices.

This approach was first described as 'tinnitus retraining therapy' in the mid 90s (Hazell, 1996). Criticism was soon evident, initially pointing out that white noise when transformed by the human ear canal and by a hearing loss no longer exhibited the flat frequency characteristics defining it as 'white' (Baguley et al., 1997), followed by critiques of the fundamental premises of the counselling technique (Wilson et al., 1998; Kröner-Herwig et al., 2000). A significant proportion of the writing about tinnitus retraining therapy has not been published in scientific journals, but instead has appeared in conference proceedings. It would not be fair to exclude this rich source of information, but as proceedings papers are scrutinized by the peer review process to a lesser degree, less weight can be put on these sources. Also, the theories and implementation of tinnitus retraining therapy have evolved somewhat since its initial conception. Therefore it would seem prudent to concentrate on the later, and presumably evolutionarily more advanced, works.

It is important to recognize that many clinicians offer a management strategy that they call tinnitus retraining therapy because it is to a greater or lesser extent based on the neurophysiological model. However, in many cases the therapeutic process does not adhere to the principles espoused by Jastreboff and Hazell: there is a difference between the neurophysiological model and its clinical implementation as tinnitus retraining therapy. Because of these terminological inexactitudes, tinnitus retraining therapy is sometimes criticized unfairly, when the treatment that is being performed is not true tinnitus retraining therapy.

Clinical protocol of tinnitus retraining therapy

Whilst tinnitus retraining therapy proponents often assert that it has not changed since its inception, publications since 1995 have elaborated and expanded the protocol and have clarified the associated terminology. In particular, the early use of 'cognitive therapy' to describe directive counselling ceased entirely (Jastreboff, 1999). The current definition of tinnitus retraining therapy consists of two elements: directive counselling and sound therapy. The only means by which one can become a formal tinnitus retraining therapy practitioner is to attend a training course with one of the originators (Henry et al., 2002, Jastreboff and Jastreboff, 2003). Although this does little to reassure one about the independence of validation studies, it does ensure purity of clinical practice. Research on tinnitus retraining therapy has not been conducted following a published structured manual, and it is often claimed that the papers describing tinnitus retraining therapy are insufficient for its implementation (Jastreboff and Jastreboff, 2000). A full manual is now available and it is hoped that this will foster more rigorous and replicable research (Jastreboff and Hazell, 2004).

A detailed history is taken of tinnitus and hyperacusis, taking appropriate steps to identify and treat those patients who require specific surgical or medical intervention (Chapter 4). Formal tinnitus retraining therapy-based questionnaires are available for this purpose (Henry et al., 2002b), facilitating a standardized, structured interview and enabling the subsequent allocation into tinnitus categories. Suitable audiological assessments are also conducted, including pure tone audiometry from 125 Hz to 8000 Hz, estimation of loudness discomfort levels over the same frequency range and tympanometry. However, in contrast to masking treatment, assessment of residual inhibition is not recommended (Henry et al., 2002b). The patient is then identified as belonging to one of five categories (Jastreboff and Jastreboff, 2003) (Table 12.1).

Table 12.1 Patient categories and suggested instrumentation, based on Jastreboff and Jastreboff (2003)

Category	Instrumentation
Category 0: Tinnitus weak or short lasting	No instruments
Category 1: Bothersome tinnitus	Sound generators
Category 2: Tinnitus and hearing loss	Combination instruments or hearing aids
Category 3: Hyperacusis with or without tinnitus:	
Without hearing loss	Sound generators
With hearing loss	Combination instruments, or sound generators followed by hearing aids
Category 4: Hyperacusis or tinnitus with sound-induced exacerbation	Sound generators or combination instruments

Patients in Category 0 do not have tinnitus with a severe impact, and treatment is titrated to that, involving counselling and the use of environmental sound for sound enrichment. Category 1 patients receive retraining counselling (Jastreboff, 1998) and ear-level sound generators set with their output below but close to the perceived tinnitus intensity. This point, where the external sound source and the tinnitus appear to be at the same level, is referred to as the 'mixing point'. Patients in Category 2 have a hearing loss in addition to tinnitus, though the level at which such an associated hearing loss becomes clinically relevant has not been clearly defined. Category 2 patients are treated with hearing aids or combination instruments, which incorporate a hearing aid and a wide-band sound generator, in conjunction with counselling. Categories 3 and 4 include patients with hyperacusis, either without or with marked exacerbation on sound exposure, respectively, and are treated with a desensitizing programme of sound (see Table 12.1), with an appropriate protocol for each category.

A somewhat expanded version of this categorization was presented by Henry et al. (2002a). Unfortunately, neither the categorization nor the structured interview has been validated scientifically, which is essential if the tinnitus retraining therapy interview is to be utilized by the wider tinnitus community. In contrast, as reviewed in Chapter 6, there are a few validation studies on structured interviews with tinnitus patients. The difficulties performing categorization as part of tinnitus retraining therapy was acknowledged by Jastreboff and Jastreboff (2003: 331), who wrote: 'The previously mentioned categories provide general approach guidance, and patients might be on the border of two categories.' However, the approach taken to categorize patients is a welcome initiative in the tinnitus community. Tinnitus retraining therapy recognizes that categorization can change during the natural history of the patient's condition or during the therapeutic management process. Thus it is important to regularly re-evaluate each patient, as a change of category may require a change of treatment plan.

The specific treatment given to each patient is detailed below, but common to all is the element of directive counselling involving teaching about 'the physiology of the auditory system. The basic principles of brain function with focus on the mechanisms of perception, attention and emotions, the role of the autonomic nervous system; and the mechanism behind creating and retraining conditioned reflexes' (Jastreboff, 1998: 92). This introduction to auditory neuroscience can be time consuming and the expertise required is considerable. When it is done well, directive counselling helps to educate the patient, which, in turn, helps to demystify tinnitus and hence to remove negative associations with tinnitus. The use of sound therapy alone without directive counselling is not sufficient (Jastreboff and Jastreboff, 2000), demonstrating that the counselling is a vital component of tinnitus retraining therapy.

In tinnitus retraining therapy the use of sound devices is not obligatory, but sound input is necessary to achieve habituation (Jastreboff and Jastreboff, 2000). Unsurprisingly, therefore, sound generators are used in most cases, with 70% being fitted with an instrument from a restricted range of sound generators approved by Jastreboff (Jastreboff, 2000; Henry et al., 2002b). Devices are always fitted bilaterally according to the guidelines produced by Jastreboff (2000), and should have open ear moulds (Henry et al., 2002b) to avoid occluding the ear canal and creating a conductive hearing loss. When using sound generators in the management of tinnitus the volume is adjusted to the mixing point at the beginning of the day, and is then not touched for the rest of the day. When using sound generators for categories 3 or 4 patients with significant hyperacusis, different instructions are issued. These patients are advised to set their sound generator to a level that is always just audible. Therefore, as the environmental noise levels fluctuate the patient needs to regularly readjust the output level of their devices. Instructions are given to use the sound generators for at least eight hours per day, or hearing aids (including combination units) for all waking hours. All patients undergoing tinnitus retraining therapy are advised to avoid silence and to enrich their sound environment. This can include all means of auditory stimulation, such as bedside sound machines, music, water features, wind chimes and so on (Jastreboff, 2000). It is also recommended that patients should have an enriched sound environment during the night (Jastreboff and Jastreboff, 2003). The tinnitus retraining therapy protocol requires that the patient adheres to the regimen for 12–24 months, and specifically, points out that habituation is a long-term process (Jastreboff et al., 1996). Regular follow-up appointments are recommended (Jastreboff and Jastreboff, 2003).

Evidence of efficacy

Peer-reviewed randomized placebo-controlled trial evidence of tinnitus retraining therapy is not present in the medical literature, though this criticism is perhaps unjustified as it is difficult to envisage how such a trial could ever be undertaken. In the absence of placebo-controlled trials, studies should utilize an untreated waiting list group, or use another established treatment as comparator. The closest treatment modality to tinnitus retraining therapy to use for comparison is psychological treatment (Chapter 13).

Observing measurements before and after treatment without a suitable control group is not a good alternative, but so far this is the main design used in studies on tinnitus retraining therapy. Evidence is emergent, however, in the form of observational studies, and it is hoped that waiting list control studies will soon appear. Previously, advocates of tinnitus retraining therapy have been somewhat antagonistic to calls for robust evidence of efficacy, invoking 'evidence by consensus' (Jastreboff and Jastreboff, 2001), meaning that methods may be demonstrated to be 'valid only when replicable and accepted by the scientific community' (Jastreboff and Jastreboff, 2001: 59). This sentiment runs contrary to evidence-based medicine (Sackett et al., 2000). More recently, however, an indication that formal trials are required before tinnitus retraining therapy can be widely adopted has been given by Henry et al. (2002a: 560), who acknowledged that 'The community of tinnitus researchers and clinicians does not operate by a common standard, and the tinnitus patient has almost no means to assess the validity of any claims regarding treatment efficacy.'

Studies containing evidence about the efficacy of tinnitus retraining therapy are summarized in Table 12.2. There are a number of concerns about this literature. First, the studies are observational, and have not been subject to rigorous peer review. The authors generally do not use standardized outcome measures, and the way responders have been defined is not validated in any way, so their reports of efficacy should be interpreted with caution. It is appropriate to describe the evidence base for tinnitus retraining therapy as emergent at best.

There are a few more robust trials not presented in Table 12.2 as they have been criticized for not using proper tinnitus retraining therapy. For example, Schmidtt and Kröner-Herwig (2002) compared cognitive behavioural therapy ($n = 27$) and tinnitus retraining therapy-like intervention conducted in groups ($n = 30$) with a one-session education or self-help group ($n = 20$). Participants were randomized to each condition. The results showed that cognitive behaviour therapy and their adaptation of tinnitus retraining therapy were equally effective, and good long-term effects were also seen. The authors concluded that cognitive behaviour therapy is a more cost-effective strategy, given the costs of sound generators. Other similar examples also exist (Haerkötter and Hiller, 2002), but as these treatments did not strictly meet the criteria for being considered as tinnitus retraining therapy, it is unfair to draw too many conclusions.

Evaluation of tinnitus retraining therapy

A number of criticisms of the neurophysiological model, and of tinnitus retraining therapy, have been voiced. Wilson et al. (1998) noted that written descriptions of the neurophysiological model (citing Jastreboff and Hazell, 1993) use terms such as 'attention', 'coping' and 'perception' in an ill-defined and obscure manner. They further asserted that the directive counselling component of tinnitus retraining therapy is a 'weak' form of cognitive therapy (Wilson et al., 1998), given that the explicit objective is to change beliefs. These criticisms called into question the adequacy and novelty of the Jastreboff neurophysiological model, which Wilson et al. (1998: 70) rather damned with faint praise: 'We are in broad agreement with the neurophysiological model – to state otherwise would be to refute the very basis of modern psychology'. An opposing viewpoint is that the neurophysiological model may indeed be somewhat simplistic, but this can be viewed as a positive attribute as it facilitates communication of the concepts to patients (Baguley, 2002). A more disturbing possibility is that the model is incorrect, and that there are missing links in the description of unconditioned stimuli and conditioned responses, as has been suggested by researchers in the psychological community (McKenna, 2004; Andersson, 2002a). Up to this day, the model has not been tested in human experimental research and the evidence presented is only indirect.

Further, although less cogent, criticism was forthcoming from Kröner-Herwig et al. (2000), who again criticized the neurophysiological model for lack of novelty and inadequacy, and advised caution regarding the use of tinnitus retraining therapy, described public praise for the technique as 'premature' (Kröner-Herwig et al., 2000: 77).

The directive counselling technique contains elements of persuasion and so could, in the hands of inexperienced clinicians, be misunderstood and even insensitive to the idiosyncrasies of the individual patient. The literature on tinnitus retraining therapy acknowledges the deep distress experienced by some tinnitus patients, but it does not fully nor explicitly take this into account in directive counselling. Onward appropriate, referral to other clinicians is a critical issue in tinnitus management. According to Henry et al. (2002b: 526), 'Audiologists must use their professional judgement to assess whether a tinnitus patient should be referred to a counsellor for a psychological or psychiatric evaluation.' Clearly, this is not evidence-based advice, and more careful assessments could easily be recommended using the readily available validated self-report screening instruments.

Given the natural course of depression, and the long duration of treatment in tinnitus retraining therapy, it is plausible that at least some of the effects of tinnitus retraining therapy could be attributed to a non-specific anti-depressant effect. This would be relatively straightforward to determine in trials on tinnitus retraining therapy by the incorporation of psychiatric assessments.

The usefulness of both the neurophysiological model and tinnitus retraining therapy to clinicians is as difficult to ascertain as their relevance to patients. At its outset, the neurophysiological model represented, and still does to this day, a clinically useful synthesis of knowledge about the human auditory system and of reciprocal links with systems of reaction and emotion. It is widely taught and understood by audiologists, and its overall value appears good. Of tinnitus retraining therapy specifically, things are less clear. Henry et al. (2002b) claim that tinnitus retraining therapy is in use in over 100 centres worldwide, which is impressive until one realizes that there are approximately 240 audiology centres in the UK alone. Thus, the adoption of tinnitus retraining therapy in pure form is not wide, and the insistence that one can practise tinnitus retraining therapy only if trained by one of the originators is not likely to further that adoption.

Summary

The contributions of Pawel Jastreboff and Jonathan Hazell to tinnitus research and therapy have been enormous. The concept that one had to look beyond

Table 12.2 Studies on the efficacy of tinnitus retraining therapy

Authors (year)	Type of publication	*n*	Design	Outcome measure	Patients improved (%)
Jastreboff et al. (1996)	Peer-reviewed journal	>100	Observational	Not specified	83% of group fitted with noise generators (*n* not specified)
Jastreboff (1998)	Book chapter	129	Observational	20% improvement in two of: interference with activities in daily life; annoyance; or per cent of time aware of tinnitus	81.4
Bartnik et al. (1999)	Conference proceedings	120 selected from 556	Observational	One life activity resumed and 20% improvement in measures of impact, annoyance and per cent of time aware of tinnitus	77.6
Heitzmann et al. (1999)	Conference proceedings	56	Observational	Not specified	84% 'greatly improved'
Herraiz et al. (1999)	Conference proceedings	84	Directive counselling versus directive counselling and sound therapy	Visual analogue scale, Tinnitus Handicap Inventory, patient report	84.2% overall improvement on counselling alone; 93.7% improvement on patient report; 83.3% improvement on counselling and sound therapy

Study	Publication	N	Study type	Outcome measure	Result
Jastreboff (1999)	Conference proceedings	223	Observational	20% improvement in two of: interference with activities in daily life; annoyance; or per cent of time aware of tinnitus	81
Kellerhals (1999)	Conference proceedings	120	Observational	Improvement in two life activities in tinnitus retraining interviews	71
McKinney et al. (1999)	Conference proceedings	182	–	40% improvement in two of: measures of annoyance; life quality; or per cent of time aware of tinnitus intensity	83.3
Sheldrake et al. (1999)	Conference proceedings	224	Observational	40% improvement in measures of annoyance and awareness; or 0% improvement in measures of annoyance and awareness, and improvement in one activity of daily life	83.7
Bartnik et al. (2001)	Journal supplement	108	Observational	'A special questionnaire'	70% of a group with tinnitus alone improved; 90% of a group with tinnitus and hearing loss
Berry et al. (2002)	Peer reviewed journal	32	Observational	Tinnitus Handicap Inventory	Statistically significant improvement

the classical auditory system, or indeed the cochlea, for an understanding of tinnitus was radical for many in the field. This change of viewpoint has had a lasting impact upon both professional and public knowledge about tinnitus. The neurophysiological model has now been utilized in teaching many audiologists, and has been widely applied to tinnitus therapy. The longer-term contribution of tinnitus retraining therapy is hard to determine at the present time, and may be somewhat constrained by an insistence that trainees should be taught about tinnitus retraining therapy only by its originators. However, there is the potential for clinicians and researchers with a holistic and neuroscientific-based understanding of tinnitus to build upon these foundations to the benefit of patients and clinicians alike.

Chapter 13
A cognitive behavioural treatment programme

Cognitive behaviour therapy is a psychological treatment approach directed at identifying and modifying unhelpful behaviours, and thoughts or cognitions (Barlow, 2001). Cognitive behaviour therapy rests on a model of psychological distress that underscores the importance of thinking or cognition and emotion. The therapeutic relation between therapist and patient in cognitive behaviour therapy is collaborative in the sense that an outline of each session and the treatment as a whole are negotiated; the therapeutic process aims to equip patients with the tools to deal with their problems rather than regarding them as passive recipients of treatment. Motivation to change habits and to alter behaviour is crucial, and it is made clear to the patient that work is required for the treatment to have any effect. The focus is on applying behavioural and cognitive techniques in real-life settings, and cognitive behaviour therapy often involves testing out coping strategies when facing difficult situations. The efficacy of cognitive behaviour therapy for psychological conditions such as anxiety and depression has been clearly demonstrated (Persons et al., 2001); the approach has also been found to be effective in the management of patients afflicted with somatic conditions, such as chronic pain (Philips and Rachman, 1996) and insomnia (Morin, 1993). The value of cognitive behaviour therapy in these other areas provides an inspiration for its application to tinnitus.

The cognitive-behavioural treatment model and its rationale

The cognitive behaviour therapy approach to tinnitus management is based on a cognitive-behavioural model of tinnitus that has been outlined by several authors (Henry and Wilson, 2001; Andersson, 2002b; Kröner-Herwig et al., 2003), but the first steps were taken by British psychologist Richard Hallam. Some early work was also conducted, by Scott and colleagues (1985) in Sweden and by Sweetow (1995) in the USA. The former group, however, had a strong behavioural emphasis in their work. The model proposed by Hallam et al. (1984) provides the main source of inspiration for the use of cognitive behaviour therapy in the management of tinnitus patients. Their psychological model of tinnitus (see Chapter 5) suggested that the natural history of tinnitus is characterized by the process of habituation. In seeking to understand tinnitus it is therefore important to investigate factors that impede habituation, for example, arousal and novelty. The model suggests that psychological treatment should focus on reducing patients' arousal and on changing the emotional significance of the tinnitus. A stress–diathesis model has been proposed for understanding the severity of tinnitus (Schulman, 1995; Andersson and McKenna, 1998) and is used in clinical practice. This suggests that the strength of the stress interacts with the person's vulnerability to stress. For example, a 'vulnerable' person might develop tinnitus distress following the onset of relatively 'mild' tinnitus, whereas a more stress-tolerant person might bear louder tinnitus before seeking help. Vulnerability does not equal 'psychiatric disturbances', but can result in all sorts of stresses in life, including somatic conditions that may exist before the onset of tinnitus.

The model proposed by Hallam et al. (1984) stresses the central role of beliefs in the distress experienced by tinnitus patients. Thoughts and beliefs about tinnitus are important and can strengthen the association between negative emotions and tinnitus. The meaning attached to tinnitus influences how annoying it is perceived to be. Many tinnitus patients report difficulties with concentration. Hence it can be suspected that tinnitus 'demands attention'. When using cognitive behaviour therapy in the treatment of tinnitus an effort is made to help the patient to accept tinnitus and to adopt the attitude that it is not worth all the attention it gets (Andersson and Kaldo, in press). Patients are helped to distinguish between useless attempts to try to control something that cannot be controlled (as often is the case with loudness of tinnitus), and successful ways of controlling reactions and emotions when faced with difficulties (e.g. the consequences of tinnitus).

A treatment package based on the cognitive behaviour therapy approach is outlined in Table 13.1. It is usually presented in six to 10 sessions on a weekly basis. Although individual treatment often is required, cognitive behaviour therapy can also be successfully used in a small group setting with tinnitus patients (Kröner-Herwig et al., 1995). Homework assignments are necessary for the treatment to make a difference in the patient's life. As the treatment focuses on the ways in which tinnitus affects everyday activities, such as work, family and leisure activities, it is important to obtain information about these areas and to encourage the patient to try out the skills taught in therapy in these relevant situations. Another important aspect of the treatment is the simple notion that 'What is good for life in general, is usually good for your ability to cope with tinnitus'. This includes living a healthy life, with respect to food, exercise, social contacts, etc. One related aspect is that it may be important for the tinnitus patient to establish regular routines in life. Before the onset of tinnitus, it might have been possible to have irregular working hours and sleep patterns, but often adaptation to tinnitus requires regular habits, in particular when it comes to maintaining sleep. As the effects of psychological treatment of tinnitus are most apparent directly after the treatment, it is crucial to schedule follow-up visits, for example at three months after the end of treatment, to assess tinnitus distress at this point. Follow-up sessions are also used to summarize the treatment, and to encourage continued use of treatment strategies, in order to prevent a return of tinnitus distress.

Table 13.1 Overview of a cognitive-behavioural treatment programme (not all aspects will apply to every clinical situation)

Structured clinical interview

Treatment rationale and information

Treatment

Applied relaxation (progressive relaxation, short progressive relaxation, cue-controlled relaxation and rapid relaxation)

Positive imagery, sound enrichment by means of external sounds, hearing tactics and advice about noise sensitivity

Modification of negative thoughts and beliefs

Behavioural sleep management

Advice about concentration difficulties, exercises of concentration (mindfulness) and physical activity

Relapse prevention

Questionnaire assessment

Follow-up (personal interview)

Psychological assessment

At least one medical consultation including audiological tests should precede the first meeting with the patient who is referred for cognitive behaviour therapy. Then the cognitive-behaviour therapist interviews the patient using a structured interview including questions on tinnitus history and characteristics, psychological and physical consequences (e.g. sleep disturbance), exacerbating and relieving factors, related symptoms and previous treatments (see Chapter 6). Typically, 1.5 hours is needed to interview the patient. The aim of the interview is to establish good therapeutic contact and to collect enough information in order to be able to decide if the patient is suitable, or not, for psychological treatment. This is typically done in the format of a functional analysis (Sturmey, 1996), which for tinnitus involves collecting information about factors that influence the tinnitus annoyance, and investigating causal links between the things that the patient does and experiences, and how tinnitus is perceived. In this first session a rationale is presented that incorporates the idiosyncrasies of the patient and also gives some preliminary goals of the treatment (McKenna, 1987). The end result of the interview can be expressed in terms of a case formulation where the major problems, goals and obstacles are presented (Persons and Davidson, 2001). The case formulation can later be revisited with new information, from self-report questionnaires, for example, supplementing the information obtained in the interview (see Chapter 6).

Applied relaxation

Applied relaxation is a set of methods by which the patient is gradually taught to relax quickly and to use self-control over bodily and mental sensations (Öst, 1987). The purpose of relaxation is to deal with the consequences of tinnitus and not to reduce tinnitus loudness (for detailed description see Andersson and Kaldo, in press). It is important to point this out at an early stage, as the patient who expects a reduction in tinnitus loudness is likely to be disappointed. There are some patients for whom applied relaxation does decrease tinnitus loudness, and such experiences should of course not be dismissed as irrelevant. It should be noted, however, that the opposite can happen initially, with temporary increases in loudness when learning relaxation. Experience suggests that it is best to prepare the patient that the most likely outcome is no change in loudness. Interestingly, there are cases in which a clear association with loudness and tension is observed, supporting the somatic modulation hypothesis of tinnitus (Cacace, 2003).

Applied relaxation can be compared to any other skill, such as learning to swim, ride a bike or drive a car, in that it takes time and practice to learn, but once it has been mastered it can be used everywhere. The goal is to obtain a relaxed physical state and a relaxed state of mind, and so to break the vicious circle of tension leading to more focus on tinnitus. Learning applied relaxation training is usually the first task that the patient is assigned in the treatment protocol described in Uppsala and in London. Although other cognitive behaviour therapy clinicians (e.g. Henry and Wilson, 2001) do not use relaxation techniques to the same extent as the UK and Swedish psychologists, proponents argue that it has considerable face validity in tinnitus management and represents an easily learnt sense of control for patients. The technique is taught in stages over four to six sessions, and the last stage is practised for the rest of the treatment once it is mastered. Usually, four components are included:

- Progressive relaxation (tense and release body parts).
- Release-only relaxation without tension.
- Cue-controlled relaxation (controlled breathing).
- Rapid relaxation in everyday situations.

Imagery techniques are taught in association with the relaxation training. Although there are few studies on the differential effects of different forms of relaxation for tinnitus (see Chapter 11), there are indications that the combination of elements of applied relaxation is slightly superior to other alternatives such as progressive relaxation (Davies et al., 1995).

Distraction and focusing

The use of attention-diversion techniques, imagery by using 'inner pictures' and exercises directly aimed at reinterpreting tinnitus as something less painful (Hallam, 1989; Henry and Wilson, 2001) form part of the treatment protocol. The goal is for the patient to learn these techniques in the clinic and then to apply the skills in real-life settings. Exposure techniques, inspired by the principles used in the treatment of phobias (Öst, 1997), are also often included. Recently these techniques have been used with chronic pain patients (Linton et al., 2002), and it appears that they may be applicable for a proportion of tinnitus patients. Strong emotional reactions, particularly involving fear and avoidance, are sometimes associated with tinnitus. They can lead to a negative view of tinnitus and can occasionally develop into panic-like attacks when the patient seeks to escape from tinnitus. Apart from advice about sound enrichment, the programme deals with adverse reactions to silence (when this is a problem) and this is an instance where exposure techniques can be helpful. A list of distraction techniques was recommended by Henry and Wilson (2001). For example, one such technique is 'thought stopping', which involves deliberate attempts to suppress thoughts about tinnitus. As stated by Henry and Wilson (2001), the idea is not so much to stop thinking about the tinnitus as it is to learn to direct attention both to and from the tinnitus. It is questionable if this works in the long term, and, theoretically, it could even be counterproductive (Wegner, 1994). In the short term, however, there is evidence to suggest that it can be a helpful strategy.

Problems with concentration are often a source of great distress for the tinnitus sufferer, and are targeted in the treatment. Methods for improving concentration and memory training have been developed by neuropsychologists (Wilson, 1987). The techniques involve structuring material to ensure encoding (e.g. to focus on one element at a time), elaboration (thinking things over, maybe using notes) and retrieval of information (e.g. using hints to aid memory). As yet these techniques have not been evaluated systematically with tinnitus patients.

Sound enrichment

Sound enrichment and attitude towards masking, partial masking, silence and fluctuations in environmental sounds constitute important parts of the treatment. This element was introduced following the development of tinnitus retraining therapy (Jastreboff, 2000), but in cognitive behaviour therapy specific tinnitus instruments, such as sound generators, are rarely used. Sound enrichment can include analysis of sound environments in the patient's daily life, tapes or CDs, but more importantly, advice and analysis of fluctuations in tinnitus loudness and explanation of the risks associated with trying to mask (i.e. cover) the tinnitus. Thoughts and beliefs in relation to sounds are an integral part of the cognitive therapy component of the treatment. For example, selective attention is described and exemplified by illustrating that tinnitus can either be masked or be made very noticeable in the same environment, depending on whether attention is directed towards or away from it (Andersson, 2002a).

Sleep management

Sleep hygiene, bedtime and worry-time restriction, relaxation and cognitive restructuring can be helpful for patients with sleep problems (McKenna, 2000; McKenna and Daniel, in press). These methods are tailored according to the special needs of the tinnitus patient. Obviously, sleep management in the case of tinnitus must include the role of sounds and how to handle wake-ups. In general, psychological treatment of insomnia often consists of stimulus-control techniques (such as going to bed only when tired, and/or getting up at the same time every day), sleep restriction (e.g. staying in bed only for expected sleep period rather than lying in), relaxation techniques, sleep hygiene and cognitive behaviour therapy programmes. The latter often combines approaches such as stimulus-control and cognitive restructuring (Morin et al., 1999). An example of a comprehensive sleep management programme is outlined in Table 13.2. Briefer consultations, however, may also be beneficial for some patients (Hauri, 1993), and sleep management is a field for which self-help methods have been successfully applied (Mimeault and Morin, 1999). Two meta-analyses have documented the effects of stimulus-control therapy, sleep restriction, relaxation and a number of different educational and cognitive strategies (Morin et al., 1994; Murtagh and Greenwood, 1995). Compared with pharmacological treatment protocols, studies have shown that non-pharmacological interventions are perceived as not only more acceptable, but they also produce more lasting improvements (Morin et al., 1999). The efficacy of multi-component approaches has been found to give slightly better result than single-component treatments (Morin et al., 1999). To date, there is no controlled outcome study of insomnia management specifically targeted towards tinnitus patients with insomnia.

Table 13.2 Components of a sleep management programme

Week 1:	Information about insomnia and sleep. Introduction to sleep restriction and stimulus control strategy I.
Week 2:	Sleep restriction and stimulus control strategies II–VI. Information about sleep medication.
Week 3:	Sleep restriction and stimulus control strategies continued. Information on negative automatic thoughts and introduction to cognitive restructuring.
Week 4:	Sleep restriction and stimulus control strategies continued. Further elaboration on cognitive techniques.
Week 5:	Sleep restriction and stimulus control strategy repetition. Continued use of cognitive restructuring techniques. Information about sleep hygiene. Relapse prevention.

Hearing tactics

The field of hearing tactics deals with different ways of facilitating communication, such as optimizing signals and using conversational strategies (Brooks, 1989). A cognitive-behavioural adaptation of hearing tactics has been developed (Andersson, 2000a) and has been found to have positive results in controlled trials (Andersson et al., 1995b). It is important to note that hearing tactics do not represent an alternative to hearing aid fitting but, rather, should be viewed as one of many ways to assist the hearing-impaired person. A condensed form of hearing tactics is commonly used in tinnitus treatments; the key features are as follows: communication skills training, in which the participant is encouraged to focus on one person and concentrate on communication with that individual. This includes proper positioning in relation to the other person, moderately expressive body language and being active in the conversation. When hearing fails, repair strategies are practised (Tye-Murray, 1991), including ways of handling missing information and asking for confirmation if the participant has understood things correctly. This necessitates active listening and focusing on meaning instead of the details of the message. Assertive responses are practised, such as informing others about the hearing loss and anticipating their reactions. Moreover, waiting for your turn, reinforcing the behaviour of the communication partner and the advantages of talking on a topic about which you have knowledge are highlighted. Distribution of a leaflet with advice on communication with hearing-impaired people that is to be presented to the closest ones (relatives) is set as a homework assignment. The role of relatives and the ways they can help, is further discussed (e.g. social skills needed).

Cognitive therapy

Cognitive restructuring of thoughts and beliefs associated with tinnitus is a central and necessary feature of cognitive behaviour therapy with tinnitus patients. Patients are helped to identify the content of their thoughts and are taught ways to challenge or control those thoughts that are unhelpful, or even inaccurate. It is important to note that this is not equal to 'positive thinking'. Some patients find the cognitive model difficult to understand at first, and it is therefore crucial that time is taken to educate them and to check that the model is understood properly. As with many other physical symptoms, tinnitus can be accompanied by negative beliefs that are not necessarily irrational. On the surface, beliefs such as 'I have tinnitus', 'It will never go away' or 'I shall never hear silence again' are reasonably accurate. Although the beliefs first expressed can be correct, it is sometimes the case that more catastrophic beliefs exist in the background. This can be in the form of 'I shall never be able to enjoy life again' or 'Tinnitus affects me very badly; I must be a very weak person'. Such unrealistic beliefs are targeted by cognitive therapy (Persons et al., 2001). It is common practice to combine the challenging of unrealistic beliefs with education about the natural course of tinnitus and a comprehensive assessment of quality of life in general. The truth is that most patients have at least a part of their life that is not affected by tinnitus. But the clinician needs to identify and distinguish irrational beliefs from accurate ones, and in particular to be careful not to go too fast when evoking thoughts (e.g. core beliefs) that might be very distressing for the patient to discover. For many patients, it is relatively straightforward to discover the content of their beliefs about tinnitus.

Relapse prevention

Relapse prevention includes a discussion of risk factors for developing more severe tinnitus and hearing loss, and devising a plan for what to do should the tinnitus become worse (Henry and Wilson, 2001). High-risk situations may also involve psychosocial aspects, such as work-related problems and marital difficulties. As part of the secondary prevention, the importance of regular practice of therapeutic techniques is covered. During treatment, or immediately afterwards, tinnitus can become temporarily louder and more noticeable. This effect, however, is often temporary and the beneficial effects of treatment always outweigh the small fluctuation in loudness the patient may perceive. One crucial aspect of cognitive behaviour therapy is to foster generalization from the treatment setting to the daily life of the patient. One way to secure continued treatment gains is to refer to matters of everyday life during treatment and to discuss how the patient can use the skills taught in treatment in different settings in life (e.g. on holiday). Lastly, one way to prevent relapse is to make sure that the patient is not abandoned once treatment has ended. Therefore the plan should include identifying whom to contact if the annoyance increases again.

Self-help and the Internet

For many conditions, such as headache, sleep problems and anxiety, there is strong support for the use of self-help materials. Self-help books can be a good alternative when professional therapy is inaccessible or is considered too expensive. Although numerous such books are available, only a fraction of them have been tested in empirical studies (Norcross et al., 2000), but, overall, self-help is well validated in outcome trials (Scogin et al., 1990). Studies of self-help treatments usually include some form of contact with the therapist, for example by means of telephone calls. Although many tinnitus sufferers seek help outside medical settings (such as the Internet), until recently researchers have paid little attention to the idea of alleviating tinnitus distress via self-help material. One way to provide self-help material in a structured manner is via the Internet (Andersson and Kaldo-Sandström, 2003). Providing treatment via the Internet has advantages over self-help books in that advice can be given on a continuous basis without delay. In comparison with ordinary treatment it is cost-effective, and it also makes the treatment available to people living far from the specialist centre.

The implementation of cognitive behaviour therapy via the Internet was initially made without any major revisions (Andersson et al., 2002b), but certain issues must be detailed to avoid misunderstanding the purpose of Internet-based self-help as it has been implemented in Uppsala, Sweden. All patients clearly need to have access to a computer, a modem and an Internet connection, and should be able to print out the training instructions. Although it is possible to go through all the steps without any personal contact, in clinical practice the patient is seen for a first assessment session, and later on for a follow-up; there are ethical and medico-legal problems associated with treating patients that have not been assessed in a clinic. All registration forms and rating scales are converted into web pages and are filled out via the Internet. Web pages are not 'open', and are only accessible with a password, given by e-mail to the patient. In cases when the Internet fails to work, or when patients have problems with their connection, the therapist can be contacted by telephone. The programme is set up in six separate modules (or weeks) that basically mirror the face-to-face treatment described previously. All modules involve homework assignments and reports on a web page, to be submitted weekly. Patients are encouraged to ask questions about the treatment and all queries are answered as promptly as possible by the therapist or the physician. An example of a web page is given in Figure 13.1.

When submitting a week's report the patient is sent an encouraging e-mail, with the instruction to go to the next module (and is given the code to that module). Some automatic processing of reports is possible, but it is generally recommended that the clinician should read all the submitted material from the patient. In the latest version of the treatment patients are encouraged to plan their treatment. Some ingredients, such as applied relaxation, are

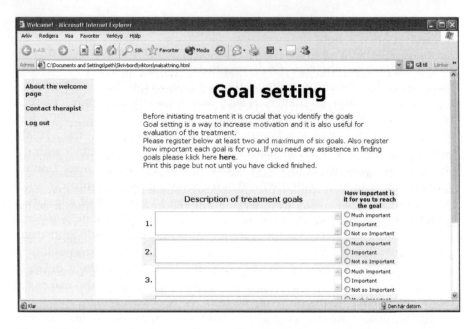

Figure 13.1 An example of a web page used in self-help for tinnitus via the Internet.

obligatory, whereas others, including hearing tactics and sleep management, are selected depending on the unique needs of each patient. In order for the programme to have any effect, it is crucial that patients go through all the appropriate exercises and that they contact the therapist if there are any questions or technical problems.

Evidence base for cognitive behaviour therapy

Cognitive behaviour therapy is among the most, if not *the* most, thoroughly validated treatment approach to tinnitus (Andersson et al., 1995c). However, there is still a lack of large-scale studies, with the exception of trials conducted in Australia by Henry and Wilson (2001). Meta-analysis is a technique of combining results from different trials in order to obtain estimates of effects across studies (Egger and Davey Smith, 1997). Two meta-analyses have been published on the effects of cognitive behaviour therapy for tinnitus (Andersson and Lyttkens, 1999; Schilter et al., 2000), showing similar results. In the meta-analysis by Schilter et al. (2000), however, the effect sizes for pharmacological studies were found to be slightly higher (Cohen's d = 1.27) compared with the psychological studies (Cohen's d = 0.88). The effect size, Cohen's d, is a standardized difference between groups or within groups (Cohen, 1988). A positive effect size indicates that the treatment group achieved better outcomes than the control group (or post-treatment improved over pre-treatment). An effect size of 0.20 is considered small, 0.50 is considered medium and 0.80 is considered large for clinical research (Cohen, 1988).

The outcomes of 18 studies of psychological treatments were summarized by Andersson and Lyttkens (1999). Their meta-analysis included a total of 24 samples and up to 700 subjects. Studies on cognitive behaviour therapy (e.g. Scott et al., 1985), relaxation (e.g. Davies et al., 1995), hypnosis (e.g. Attias et al., 1993), biofeedback (e.g. Haralambous et al., 1987), educational sessions (e.g. Dineen et al., 1997b) and problem solving (e.g. Wise et al., 1998) were all included. Effect sizes for perceived tinnitus loudness, annoyance, negative affect (such as depression) and sleep problems were calculated for randomized controlled studies, pre–post design studies and follow-up results. The results showed strong to moderate effects on tinnitus annoyance for controlled studies (Cohen's $d = 0.86$), pre–post designs (Cohen's $d = 0.50$) and at follow-up (Cohen's $d = 0.48$). The results on tinnitus loudness were weaker and disappeared at follow-up. Lower effect sizes were also obtained for measures of negative affect and sleep problems. Exploratory analyses revealed that cognitive behaviour therapy (Cohen's $d = 1.1$) was more effective than other psychological treatments (Cohen's $d = 0.30$) on ratings of annoyance in the controlled studies.

One potentially crucial aspect of cognitive behaviour therapy for tinnitus is its long-term effect. Although Andersson and Lyttkens (1999) found some evidence for long-term results, closer inspection of the controlled trials has not supplied proof of positive long-term outcome. In a recent trial by Henry and Wilson (unpublished data); however, results were impressive and indeed stable across the 12-month follow-up. In a non-controlled study, Andersson et al. (2001) collected longitudinal data for an average period of five years after cognitive behaviour therapy, showing decreases in annoyance and an increase in tolerance of tinnitus.

In clinical psychology research it has become useful practice to calculate the proportion of clients showing a clinical significant improvement following treatment (Ogles et al., 2001). This is often defined as a 50% decrease on the outcome measure of interest (Blanchard and Schwartz, 1988) and should be distinguished from statistical significance, which often reflects much more modest improvement. In a recent study, Henry and Wilson (unpublished data) reported that more than 70% of their patients reached this clinically significant criterion on the Tinnitus Reaction Questionnaire. In most other studies, the proportion of significantly improved tinnitus patients has not been reported. It is, however, unlikely to be as high as 70%. On average, an estimation of the effects of cognitive behaviour therapy in clinical practice is that about 30–50% of patients improve significantly. As stated above, the effect of cognitive behaviour therapy on insomnia in relation to tinnitus has not been investigated in any depth. Clinical experience attests to the usefulness of sleep management (McKenna, 2000; McKenna and Daniel, in press), but in the meta-analysis only two controlled studies were identified in which sleep problems had been measured before and after treatment (Jakes et al., 1992; Kröner-Herwig et al., 1995). Andersson et al. (2002b) collected diary recordings in an Internet-based study but found no effects on insomnia. More recently, Kaldo et al. (2004) found significant reductions on the Insomnia Severity Index (Bastien et al., 2001), suggesting that sleep can improve after cognitive behaviour therapy for tinnitus.

There are few CB therapists working in the field of tinnitus and therefore this form of therapy can be difficult to access. There has been some recent interest in the idea of minimal therapist contact and self-help treatments. For example, Kröner-Herwig et al., (2003) found that two minimal contact interventions resulted in positive results with reductions in disability. In a recent unpublished randomized controlled trial on the benefits of a self-help book (cognitive behaviour therapy-based) in combination with weekly telephone calls, significant improvements were found – suggesting that assisted self-help could also be a treatment alternative.

Three trials on the effects of Internet-based self-help treatment have been conducted. In the first study (Andersson et al., 2002a), participants were recruited through web pages and newspaper articles, and they were then randomly allocated to a cognitive behaviour therapy self-help manual in six modules, or to a waiting list control group. All treatment and contact with participants was conducted via the Internet with web pages and e-mail correspondence. The participants were 117 people with tinnitus of at least six months' duration. In the first phase of the study 26 subjects completed all stages of treatment (49%) and 64 subjects from the waiting list control group provided measures. At one-year follow-up all participants had been offered the programme, and 96 provided outcome measures, yielding an 18% dropout rate from baseline to follow-up. Tinnitus-related problems were assessed before and after treatment, and at the one-year follow-up. Daily diary-ratings were included for one week before and one week after the treatment period. Results showed that tinnitus-related distress, depression and diary ratings of annoyance caused by tinnitus decreased significantly. Immediately following the first study phase (with a waiting list control group), significantly more participants in the treatment group showed an improvement of 50% on the Tinnitus Reaction Questionnaire. At follow-up 27 (31%) had achieved a clinically significant improvement.

In the second Internet study, participants ($n = 77$) were recruited from an audiology clinic (Kaldo et al., 2004). The results from the first study were replicated. In order to describe in more depth what actually goes on in Internet-based treatment one case has been detailed in a case study (Andersson and Kaldo, 2004).

Lastly, in the most recent Internet study, group cognitive behaviour therapy has been compared with an updated Internet-based treatment. The patients were randomly assigned to either group treatment ($n = 23$) or to

Internet-based self-help ($n = 24$). Using clinical significant change on the Tinnitus Reaction Questionnaire as an outcome measure, 42.6% of the group patients and 43.5% of the Internet patients reached this criterion. In fact, no differences could be detected between the two groups.

Evaluation of cognitive behaviour therapy

The availability of clinical psychology services for tinnitus patients was commented on by Coles (1992). He stated that there were few clinical psychologists working with tinnitus patients in the UK, and that few patients were referred to psychiatrists or psychologists. Referring to data from a survey of tinnitus management, he noted that only nine of 458 consultants referred patients to psychiatrists or clinical psychologists more than 15 times per year. This is probably still the case today – more than 10 years later. Experiences from the field of chronic pain, however, suggests that multidisciplinary treatments can work very well (Jensen et al., 1995) and that cognitive behaviour therapy principles can be incorporated as long as the staff are trained in the provision of the methods. In principle, there seems little direct danger in audiologists and related professionals applying cognitive behaviour therapy, but perhaps the treatment will be best provided when training manuals which provide step-by-step guidance are available. Supervision by a trained cognitive behaviour therapists is another alternative, in particular for consultations regarding difficult patients. Clearly, each person dealing with tinnitus patients, either directly or via supervision, should have a fundamental knowledge about tinnitus and the auditory aspects involved. Although most patients will not need a psychologist, there are, of course, occasions when a referral is needed. Therefore, it is crucial to know when to refer to a cognitive behaviour therapist. Self-report measures such as the Hospital Anxiety and Depression Scale (see Chapter 6) can be used for initial screening, but sometimes it is necessary to refer for an assessment by a psychologist, or a psychiatrist in the case of suspected psychopathology. For less complicated cases, self-help is an alternative, in particular when support can be given by the staff in the clinic. This can be done via e-mail or telephone calls. It is likely that there will be an increased role for Internet technology in tinnitus management in the future.

There are often several different elements within any given tinnitus treatment; this is as true of cognitive behaviour therapy as of other treatment approaches. This makes it difficult to know what treatment ingredients are the most effective, which are necessary and which ones could be omitted. All forms of cognitive behaviour therapy must involves an understanding and caring therapist (even when he or she is on the other side of an Internet connection) and the importance of this in tinnitus management should not be dismissed (Tyler et al., 2001).

Summary

Cognitive behaviour therapy for tinnitus involves identifying and modifying maladaptive behaviours, thoughts and feelings by means of practical hands-on work and homework assignments. Cognitive behaviour therapy has been practised for many years, but is still not widely used in tinnitus management. This is unfortunate as research suggests that this approach benefits many patients, in particular when tinnitus is a significant source of distress in the patient's life. While there is little evidence that cognitive behaviour therapy has any long-term effects on the perceived loudness of tinnitus, the benefits regarding annoyance are clearer and have been replicated in many studies. It is desirable, however, to continue to develop and implement cognitive behaviour therapy treatments in which the criteria of clinically significant improvement are met. Other challenges involve the dissemination of cognitive behaviour therapy to a broader multidisciplinary community. Potentially, recently developed self-help approaches might facilitate such progress. Finally, cognitive behaviour therapy can be incorporated with other existing approaches to tinnitus management, such as the teaching component of tinnitus retraining therapy (Haerkötter and Hiller, 2002).

Chapter 14
Complementary medicine approaches to tinnitus

In 2003 the Royal College of Pathologists won a Silver Medal at the Chelsea Flower Show with an exhibition of plants, both healing and injurious to health, entitled 'Pathologists and Plants working in partnership'. A spokesman was quoted as saying 'Plants were the basis of all medicine at one time .. ' It is salutary to remember that present medical practice, however evidence-based, derives from folk medicine and custom. Treatments outside the medical domain should be considered with respect, as there may be effects at work that are not yet understood. As individuals, the authors of this book have each personally undertaken or had a close family member undertake a complementary therapy in good faith: as tinnitus specialists it is, however, important to critically consider available evidence of efficacy of treatments for tinnitus, and indeed their potential for harm.

Given the poor record of conventional Western medicine in treating tinnitus, it should not be surprising that many patients have sought recourse to 'complementary medicine' (this term being preferred to 'alternative medicine' as it is less pejorative). In an investigation of the treatments patients had sought before being seen by a psychologist in a tinnitus clinic in Sweden, Andersson (1997) found that of 69 consecutive patients seeking help for troublesome tinnitus, only 24 (35%) had not undertaken treatment before seeking clinical help, these treatments included acupuncture, non-specific relaxation therapy and various other complementary approaches. Analysis indicated that the non-treatment patients showed a statistically significant difference from the treatment group, in that they showed greater acceptability for change. Thus, seeking treatment outside the clinical domain may have an effect in hardening attitudes and beliefs about tinnitus, though it should be noted that the group investigated, by definition, had not benefited from their prior treatment.

When considering complementary medicine we should be mindful of the placebo effect. *Placebo* is Latin for 'I shall please'. In the Renaissance, a placebo was a fake potion or manipulation (Basmajian, 1999; Tyler et al., 2001) and the term became pejorative. The term 'placebo effect' became common with the use of controlled trials that utilize an inert substance or procedure, against which to compare the effect of potentially active treatment. However, according to many sources the placebo effect is fundamental to medical treatment, and the placebo effect is not the same as lack of an effect (Evans, 2003). The use of the term 'placebo effect' in tinnitus treatment does not do justice to the good faith in which attempts are made to improve a patient's situation (Tyler et al., 2001). Indeed, the observation made by Duckert and Rees (1984), that 40% of tinnitus patients reported an effect on their tinnitus following placebo injection, is often quoted as 'evidence' of huge placebo effects in the management of tinnitus. In reality, fluctuations of loudness may be of minimal relief for the tinnitus patient and might even be irrelevant for the annoyance experienced.

Homeopathic remedies

The use of homeopathy is widespread in both Europe and the USA (Eisenberg et al., 1998), despite the fundamental principle of homeopathic therapy being contrary to those of modern pharmacology (Vandenbroucke, 1997). Homeopathy is based upon the principle of similars, in that 'a patient with a specific pattern of symptoms is best treated by a remedy which causes the same or very similar pattern in healthy subjects' (Linde et al., 2001: 4), although the remedies are given in high dilution so that they may be 'unlikely to contain any molecules of the originally diluted agents' (Linde et al., 2001: 4). Simpson et al. (1998) undertook a well-designed and rigorous study of a homeopathic remedy entitled 'Tinnitus' and the results indicated no benefit of this homeopathic remedy for tinnitus compared with placebo. There are many homeopathic remedies for tinnitus available for sale on the Internet, none of which has been subject to controlled trial evaluation.

Acupuncture

Acupuncture involves the stimulation of defined points on the body by the insertion of needles or manual pressure (acupressure). The principle is based upon traditional Chinese medical concepts wherein the flow of energy around the body (Chi) is the basis of the patient's disorder, and that can be influenced by stimulation of a relevant point on the body (Linde et al., 2001). There have been a number of studies considering the effects of acupuncture upon tinnitus, using variable amounts of scientific rigour. The results are summarised in Table 14.1. A cautionary note should be struck about acupuncture. Not only has it been shown not to benefit tinnitus patients in previous reviews (Dobie, 1999; Park et al., 2000), but it has been demonstrated occasionally to have been a factor in the exacerbation of tinnitus (Andersson and Lyttkens, 1996), albeit of temporary nature.

Table 14.1 Investigations of the effect of acupuncture upon tinnitus

Authors (year)	Design	n	Finding
Hansen et al. (1982)	Sham control	17	No advantage over placebo
Marks et al. (1984)	Sham control	14	No advantage over placebo
Axelsson et al. (1994)	Sham control	20	No advantage over placebo
Gu and Axelsson (1996)	Observational	625	'More than 50% were helped'
Furugård et al. (1998)	Control (physiotherapy)	22	Significant improvement which fell to pre-treatment level at 12 months
Vilholm et al. (1998)	Randomized, double-blind placebo-controlled	52	No advantage over placebo
Nebeska et al. (1999)	Crossover study: placebo (laser), acupunture	16	Reduction of tinnitus intensity following acupuncture but not placebo (statistically significant)

Ginkgo biloba

Ginkgo biloba is an extract from the Chinese ginkgo tree, and has been used in Chinese medicine for thousands of years. Studies suggest that ginkgo has antihypoxic, free radical-scavenging, antioxidant, metabolic, antiplatelet and microcirculatory actions (Ernst, 2002). Holgers et al. (1994) investigated the effects of ginkgo biloba in a trial with an unusual design. First, an open study design was used in which 80 patients tried Ginkgo biloba. Then responders ($n = 21$) were recruited to a double-blind study. Interestingly, there were six patients who experienced the opposite effect and got worse. However, in the controlled phase no support for the use of Ginkgo biloba was found. The study was later criticized by Ernst and Stevinson (1999), who claimed that the Ginkgo biloba was underdosed. Instead, in their review, they described five randomized controlled trials, which they interpreted as showing that Ginkgo biloba extracts are effective in treating tinnitus. More recently, Drew and Davies (2001) conducted the largest trial on Ginkgo biloba and tinnitus, with 1121 participants. The intervention lasted for 12 weeks and consisted of either 50 mg Ginkgo biloba extract or placebo administered three times daily. Results showed no significant differences between the groups though critics of this trial have suggested that the dosage of Ginkgo biloba was below the therapeutic level. In some studies Ginkgo biloba has been combined with laser treatment, showing some promise in one uncontrolled trial (Plath and Oliver, 1995) and no effects in a placebo controlled trial (von Wedel et al., 1995).

Other complementary approaches

No study has been published on the use of St John's wort (*Hypericum perforatum*) in the treatment of tinnitus. However, given the common use of St John's wort in the treatment of depression, it could potentially be helpful for at least some tinnitus patients. Some caution is needed as this might pertain only to mild depression (Ernst, 2002), and it might be less effective for moderately severe depression (Hypericum Depression Trial Study Group, 2002). In addition, serious concern exists about its interaction with several conventional drugs such as antidepressants (Ernst, 2002).

Melatonin is a hormone secreted at night by the pineal gland, and it acts as a natural hypnotic in the regulation of the sleep–wake cycle. It is available without prescription in health food stores, in some countries. Observing the role of sleep loss in tinnitus, Rosenberg et al. (1998) undertook a controlled crossover study on its effects on tinnitus. Included were 30 patients who showed similar improvements following placebo and active treatment. However, a slight difference was found in favour of melatonin for the patients who reported insomnia related to their tinnitus.

Meditation can help in relaxation, but some forms of this are almost a cult or religion. Occasionally this can be abused and become very expensive. Tinnitus patients should avoid meditation that requires the practitioner to sit in silence. In one controlled trial of yoga, Kröner-Herwig et al. (1995) compared this form of relaxation with cognitive behavioural therapy. The trial involved 43 patients and results showed effects favouring cognitive behavioural therapy over yoga and a control condition.

Reflexology and aromatherapy, and such therapies, tend to promote a degree of relaxation and feeling of physical well-being as a form of relaxation. Thus they may indeed be very helpful for some tinnitus patients, although there are still too few investigations to confidently say anything about their efficacy.

Dietary supplements

A variety of dietary supplements have been suggested to have a beneficial effect upon tinnitus. One should bear in mind, however, that it is relatively easy to engender toxic levels of several vitamins and minerals using supplements purchased from supermarkets, health food stores or by mail order, and caution should be urged by clinicians and exercised by patients. Whilst the absence of evidence of efficacy of specific dietary supplements is detailed below, this can be summarized by saying that no remotely convincing evidence for efficacy of such agents yet exists.

The possibility that vitamin B complex supplements may be beneficial for tinnitus has been raised, and Seidman and Babu (2003) consider that vitamins B1 (thiamine), B3 (niacin), B6 (pyridoxine) and B12 (cobalamin) may have a specific role. The evidence quoted is anecdotal at best, despite the ease of conducting a placebo-controlled trial in this area.

Several minerals have been suggested as treatments for tinnitus. Shambaugh (1986) and DeBartolo (1989) proposed zinc deficiency as a mechanism of tinnitus generation, and advocated the use of supplements. Hypozincaemia was not supported as a mechanism for tinnitus, however, by Gersdorff et al. (1987), and a placebo-controlled trial of zinc supplements for tinnitus did not demonstrate benefit above placebo control (Paaske et al., 1991). Ochi et al. (1997) reported an improvement in troublesome tinnitus in a group treated with zinc supplements in an uncontrolled study, and repeated this study with a control group (Ochi et al., 2003), again eliciting data supporting the use of zinc in tinnitus treatment. Another uncontrolled study was reported to indicate benefit from zinc supplements by Yetiser et al. (2002), and a placebo-controlled trial by Arda et al. (2003) again indicated benefit. In no study, however, has benefit been shown to persist, and neither has the possibility that benefit be specific to patients with demonstrable zinc deficiency been rigorously investigated. Thus, despite several studies in this area, the observation of Ochi et al. (2003: 25) that 'the clinical correlation between zinc and tinnitus remains obscure' seems pertinent.

Reports have appeared in the UK popular press indicating that magnesium supplements may benefit individuals with troublesome tinnitus. The only evidence cited in support of this is not relevant and consists of a study by Attias et al. (1994) that tentatively suggested that magnesium supplements may reduce the risk of noise-induced hearing loss in battle combatants. Seidman and Babu (2003) supplant this evidence with anecdote, but the evidence for efficacy of magnesium supplements in tinnitus is paltry at best.

Stimulation of the ear

Direct electrical stimulation of the ear is discussed in Chapter 11. Various other forms of aural stimulation have been tried with variable success. Alternating magnetic fields have been tried, together with powerful magnets placed close to the tympanic membrane. In uncontrolled trials, high success rates have been claimed, but controlled trials have been negative (Coles et al., 1991).

Ultrasonic stimulation has been tried, with an initial suggestion of benefit (Carrick et al., 1986), but this was not repeatable (Rendell et al., 1987). Interestingly, in the initial study participants were described as 'An enthusiastic group of 40 patients' (Carrick et al., 1986: 153), but despite this observation only 28 of them completed the study.

Lasers have been tried in Germany, Austria and some other countries (Shiomi et al., 1997; Walger et al., 1998; Shiomi et al., 1997), but careful investigation by Mirz et al. (1999c) does not commend them to clinical use.

In that study, 50 patients were treated with either active or placebo low-power laser irradiation given through the external acoustic meatus of the affected ear directed towards the cochlea. The treatment was given for periods of 10 minutes per day for a total of 15 sessions, given over three weeks. Results showed only moderate improvement, with no significant differences between active laser and placebo. The authors concluded that low-power laser treatment is not indicated in the treatment of tinnitus. Nakashima et al. (2002) came to the same conclusion in a double-blind study involving 45 tinnitus patients with disabling tinnitus.

Hopi ear candles

Ear candling is a practice wherein the recipient lies on the side whilst a hollow cone that has been soaked in paraffin and has been allowed to harden is placed inside the ear and lit. Anecdotal reports of benefits for cerumen and tinnitus are available, the mechanism being said to be the creation of a vacuum in the ear canal. More formal investigation has determined, however, that not only do ear candles not produce a negative pressure within the ear canal, but also that serious harm may befall the participant (Seely et al., 1996). Specifically, burns, occlusion of the external auditory meatus with wax, and of perforation of the tympanic membrane have been documented (Seeley et al., 1996), and this has caused the Food and Drug Administration (FDA) to issue a stern cautionary alert about their use (IA 77-01, 1998).

Summary

The question remains as to whether the tinnitus therapist should encourage or discourage patients about undertaking complementary therapy. There is a common misconception that herbal medicinal products are devoid of adverse effects, which is not true (Ernst, 2002), and this is also the case for overuse of vitamin and mineral supplements. Furthermore, the effect of repeatedly trying therapy in the complementary domain may prove not only expensive, but repeatedly disappointing, with resultant demotivation. This effect was demonstrated empirically in attenders at a tinnitus clinic who had tried other treatments and who demonstrated significantly less acceptance of change and novel concepts (Andersson, 1997). Caution in the use of complementary therapy should be advised by a tinnitus therapist.

The placebo effect has been invoked repeatedly above. Tyler et al. (2001) advocate harnessing the placebo effect in tinnitus treatment, proposing the following strategy:

- Be perceived as a knowledgeable professional.
- Be sympathetic toward the patient.

- Demonstrate that you understand the problem.
- Provide a clear therapy plan.
- Show that you care.
- Provide feelings of mastery.
- Provide hope.
- Instil confidence in the tinnitus clinician.

Whilst such suggestions are neither new (Fowler, 1948) nor applicable only to tinnitus, they are of such eminently good and common sense that they are commended to tinnitus clinicians, mainstream or complementary alike.

Chapter 15
A multidisciplinary synthesis

Tinnitus has received enormous publicity during recent years, and the increased interest is of great potential benefit for the millions of individuals who are distressed by this common symptom. Activity in tinnitus research is slowly answering questions about the best way to undertake tinnitus management. Within the large number of studies that have been published, however, there are many with unique and sometimes idiosyncratic designs, so that comparison between test results or treatments is often nigh on impossible. In brief, the major problem is a lack of large-scale, well-conducted randomized controlled trials (Dobie, 1999, 2002). On a more promising note, important findings are emerging on the basic mechanisms behind the generation of tinnitus and its consequences (Baguley, 2002), and it is hoped that this bulk of new knowledge will inform treatments and lead clinicians to consider how to further develop their protocols. Although still at an early stage, there are also indications that systematic integrative meta-analyses can be conducted on the tinnitus literature (Andersson and Lyttkens, 1999; Schilter et al., 2000), which will bring order into the field of tinnitus research.

Once the acute distress of patients seen in the tinnitus clinic has passed, there is often time for reflection and wider-ranging discussion. At this point, usually at follow up appointments, patients may remark 'Why is there no research into tinnitus?' or 'Why does no one really understand this?'. The reader will by now have realized that there is much research (for instance, 5000 papers currently appear in a MEDLINE search on 'tinnitus'), and there are many models, so that the challenge facing the tinnitus clinician and researcher is the integration of these insights into a whole that is congruent with personal clinical experience and understanding.

Another common question is 'Why has there been so little progress with tinnitus?'. There are, of course, issues of financial resources and staffing levels, but one major factor has been the lack of interdisciplinary communication and collaboration. The inadequacy of any one discipline or perspective to perceive the tinnitus as a whole can be illustrated by an ancient Sufi story, retold by Senge (1990):

166

As three blind men encountered an elephant, each exclaimed aloud. 'It is a large rough thing, wide and broad, like a rug,' said the first, grasping an ear. The second, holding the trunk, said 'I have the real facts. It is a straight and hollow pipe.' And the third, holding a front leg, said 'It is mighty and firm, like a pillar.' Given these men's way of knowing, they will never know an elephant.

Thus a cellular physiologist considering tinnitus may see patterns of activity in the cochlear nerve; a psychologist may see emotional distress and cognitive distortions; an audiologist may see hearing loss; and an otologist possible aural pathology. Working effectively with tinnitus patients, both now and in the future, requires us to find new ways of knowing. In a clinical context, the perspectives of otology, audiology and psychology can work together, and in research the additional perspectives of pharmacology and neuroscience are of profound importance. It is only by working together that we can see the whole elephant and then begin to design truly effective treatment and therapeutic interventions.

There are several practical implications for this call for synthesis on a conceptual level. First, tinnitus patients will be best served clinically by being treated by a multidisciplinary team. Indeed, the notion of a multidimensional management approach to tinnitus patients is not new (Stephens et al., 1986; Coles and Hallam, 1987), but perhaps not often put into practice apart from in a few specialist centres. It is not possible to be prescriptive about the exact composition of a tinnitus team because of variations in staffing, skills and experience, both locally and globally. However, underlying this book is the principle that tinnitus patients deserve effective diagnosis by an informed and interested clinician, and that therapy should be undertaken by an experienced professional with a deep understanding of all the different perspectives of tinnitus. Furthermore, there should be clear and explicit referral paths for patients whose issues fall outside the scope of practice of the core team members.

The second implication concerns the knowledge base of the team members. It would not be appropriate to expect an otologist or an audiologist to be fully aware of all the details and practical aspects of cognitive behavioural therapy, and neither would one expect a psychologist to be fully conversant with the details of otological practice. One should expect, however, these professionals to be literate in these other disciplines, so that they are aware of the broad scope of practice and are able to integrate insights and concepts from those other disciplines into their own understanding and practice. An example of this has been the writing of this book, in that it should not be assumed that the psychological chapters were written by psychologists, and that the otology-related elements were written by an otologist or an audiologist. On the contrary, all the chapters have had a team approach, with much discussion about evidence and conceptual robustness from all disciplines.

Third, it almost goes without saying that this team approach can only be achieved by hard work and dedication, and in an atmosphere of mutual respect and positive regard (Tyler et al., 2001). Finally, it should also be noted that the above is not asking for the moon, in that such multidisciplinary treatment teams and protocols are evident in other fields, chronic pain management being an example where benefit to patients has been explicitly demonstrated (Flor et al., 1992). Brooks and Chalmers (1991), in a paper on training in audiology, presented a promising model of the core knowledge needed in audiology, and linked professional knowledge that can be attached to this core basic knowledge. Clearly, this is relevant for tinnitus management too. A tentative model is presented below (Figure 15.1), outlining what we believe should be the first line of practitioners seeing tinnitus patients, and the second tier of specialists to whom difficult clinical problems can be referred. What then should this basic core knowledge about tinnitus contain? We hope we have covered not only this basic knowledge but also a portion of information that, although not clinically essential for each professional who sees tinnitus patients, will expand their understanding of tinnitus and its consequences.

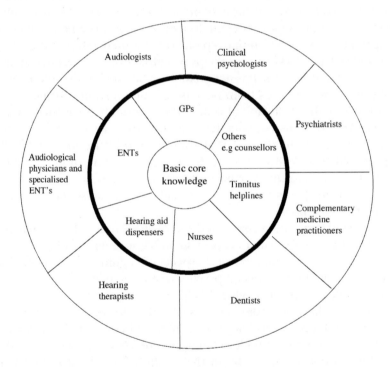

Figure 15.1 Core professional knowledge needed for tinnitus management.

Some readers, having reached this point, may have become concerned that they have not been instructed in exactly what to do or say to a tinnitus patient sitting in front of them. We believe that such a prescriptive or 'cook-book' approach is neither helpful nor respectful to the individual situation of the patient, nor indeed to the experience and skills of the clinician or therapist. In any case, such material is readily available elsewhere. It has been of more importance, we believe, to have laid out current understandings of tinnitus, incorporating theoretical and practical perspectives, so that the reader may have a wide understanding of the topic that will inform their practice.

What then of the future for tinnitus research and therapy? Baguley et al. (2003) delineated a vision for tinnitus research, wherein novel techniques and insights from neuroscience might be utilized to determine the mechanisms of tinnitus, giving targets for therapy and the means of robust determination of the efficacy of such therapy. As has been described earlier (Chapter 11) the hope for pharmacological therapy is not dead, and the prospect of integration of pharmacological treatment with counselling therapy is intriguing. The future of present therapies is also interesting to consider. Both psychological therapies and tinnitus retraining therapy are based upon conceptual models of tinnitus that are not fully satisfactory. Furthermore, the therapeutic approaches derived from these models are limited both in their application, in the case of formal psychological therapy by the number of interested psychologists available, and in tinnitus retraining therapy by the insistence on attending a formal tinnitus retraining therapy training course. What is needed is a therapeutic approach that is widely available, and based upon insights from both the psychological and neurophysiological models, which in our view are neither mutually exclusive nor immiscible. It is our hope that this book may in some small way promote such approaches and syntheses.

References

Abel SM (1990) The extra-auditory effects of noise and annoyance: an overview of research. Journal of Otolaryngology (Supp. 1): 1-13.

Adams F (1844) The Seven Books of Paulus Aeginata. London: Sydenham Society.

Allen RE (1990) Concise Oxford Dictionary of Current English. Oxford: Clarendon Press.

Alster J, Shemesh Z, Ornan M, Attias J (1993) Sleep disturbance associated with chronic tinnitus. Biological Psychiatry 34: 84-90.

American Psychiatric Association (1994) Diagnostic and Statistical Manual of Mental Disorders. Washington, DC: American Psychiatric Press.

Anari M, Axelsson A, Eliasson A, Magnusson L (1999) Hypersensitivity to sound. Questionnaire data, audiometry and classification. Scandinavian Audiology 28: 219-230.

Andersson G (1996) The role of optimism in patients with tinnitus and in patients with hearing impairment. Psychology and Health 11: 697-707.

Andersson G (1997) Prior treatments in a group of tinnitus sufferers seeking treatment. Psychotherapy and Psychosomatics 66: 107-110.

Andersson G (2000a) Hearing impairment. In: Radnitz C (ed.). Cognitive-behavioral Interventions for Persons with Disabilities. Northvale, NJ: Jason Aronson; 183-204.

Andersson G (2000b) Tinnitus: orsaker, teorier och behandlingsmöjligheter [Tinnitus. Theories, causes, and treatment options]. Lund: Studentlitteratur.

Andersson G (2000c) Longitudinal follow-up of occupational status in tinnitus patients. International Tinnitus Journal 6: 127-129.

Andersson G (2001) The role of psychology in managing tinnitus: a cognitive behavioural approach. Seminars in Hearing 22: 65-76.

Andersson G (2002a) A cognitive-affective theory for tinnitus: experiments and theoretical implications. In: Patuzzi R (ed.). Proceedings of the Seventh International Tinnitus Seminar. Freemantle: University of Western Australia; 197-200.

Andersson G (2002b) Psychological aspects of tinnitus and the application of cognitive-behavioral therapy. Clinical Psychology Review 22: 977-990.

Andersson G (2003) Tinnitus loudness matchings in relation to annoyance and grading of severity. Auris Nasus Larynx 30: 129-133.

Andersson G, Carlbring P, Kaldo V, Ström L (2004) Screening of psychiatric disorders via the Internet. A pilot study with tinnitus patients. Nordic Journal of Psychiatry 58: 287-291.

Andersson G, Eriksson J, Lundh L-G, Lyttkens L (2000c) Tinnitus and cognitive interference: a Stroop paradigm study. Journal of Speech, Hearing, and Language Research 43: 1168-1173.

171

Andersson G, Ingerholt C, Jansson M (2003a) Autobiographical memory in patients with tinnitus. Psychology and Health 18: 667-675.

Andersson G, Kaldo V (2003) Treating tinnitus via the Internet. CME Journal. Otorhinolaryngology, Head and Neck Surgery 7: 38-40.

Andersson G, Kaldo V (in press a) Cognitive-behavioral therapy with applied relaxation. In: Tyler RS (ed.). Tinnitus Treatments. Stuttgart: Thieme Publications.

Andersson G, Kaldo-Sandström V, Ström L, Strömgren T (2003) Internet administration of the hospital Anxiety and Depression Scale (HADS) in a sample of tinnitus patients, Journal of Psychosomatic Research 55: 259-262.

Andersson G, Kaldo V (2004) Internet-based cognitive behavioural therapy for tinnitus. Journal of Clinical Psychology 60: 171-178.

Andersson G, Kinnefors A, Ekvall L, Rask-Andersen H (1997) Tinnitus and translabyrinthine acoustic neuroma surgery. Audiology & Neuro-Otology 2: 403-409.

Andersson G, Lindvall N, Hursti T, Carlbring P (2002a) Hypersensitivity to sound (hyperacusis). A prevalence study conducted via the Internet and post. International Journal of Audiology 41: 545-554.

Andersson G, Lyttkens L (1996) Acupuncture for tinnitus: time to stop? Scandinavian Audiology 25: 273-275.

Andersson G, Lyttkens L (1999) A meta-analytic review of psychological treatments for tinnitus. British Journal of Audiology 33: 201-210.

Andersson G, Lyttkens L, Hirvelä C, Furmark T, Tillfors M, Fredrikson M (2000b) Regional cerebral blood flow during tinnitus: a PET case-study with lidocaine and auditory stimulation. Acta Oto-Laryngologica 120: 967-972.

Andersson G, Melin L, Lindberg P, Scott B (1995a) Development of a short scale for self-assessment of experiences of hearing impairment: the Hearing Coping Assessment. Scandinavian Audiology 24: 147-154.

Andersson G, McKenna L (1998) Tinnitus masking and depression. Audiology 37: 174-182.

Andersson G, Melin L, Scott B, Lindberg P (1995b) An evaluation of a behavioural treatment approach to hearing impairment. Behaviour Research and Therapy 33: 283-292.

Andersson G, Melin L, Hägnebo C, Scott B, Lindberg P (1995c) A review of psychological treatment approaches for patients suffering from tinnitus. Annals of Behavioral Medicine 17: 357-366.

Andersson G, Lyttkens L, Larsen HC (1999) Distinguishing levels of tinnitus distress. Clinical Otolaryngology 24: 404-410.

Andersson G, Olsson E, Rydell A-M, Larsen HC (2000a) Social competence and behaviour problems in children with hearing impairment. Audiology 39: 88-92.

Andersson G, Strömgren T, Ström L, Lyttkens L (2002b) Randomised controlled trial of Internet based cognitive behavior therapy for distress associated with tinnitus. Psychosomatic Medicine 64: 810-816.

Andersson G, Vretblad P (2000) Tinnitus and anxiety sensitivity. Scandinavian Journal of Behaviour Therapy 29: 57-64.

Andersson G, Vretblad P, Larsen H-C, Lyttkens L (2001) Longitudinal follow-up of tinnitus complaints. Archives of Otolaryngology – Head and Neck Surgery 127: 175-179.

Arda HN, Tuncel U, Akdogan O, Ozluoglu LN (2003) The role of zinc in the treatment of tinnitus. Otology Neurotology 24: 86-89.

Arnesen AR (1984) Fibre population of the vestibulocochlear anastomosis in humans. Acta Otolaryngology 98: 501-518.

Arnold W, Friedmann IJ (1988) Otosclerosis – an inflammatory disease of the otic capsule of viral aetiology. Journal of Laryngology and Otology 102: 865-871.

Arnold W, Bartenstein P, Oesstreicher E, Römer W, Schwaiger M (1996) Focal metabolic activation in the predominant left auditory cortex in patients with tinnitus: a PET study with [18F] deoxyclucose, ORL. Journal of Otorhinolaryngology Related Spec 58: 195-199.

Arts HA (1998) Differential diagnosis of sensorineural hearing loss. In: Cummings CW, Fredrickson JM, Harker LA et al. (eds). Otolaryngology Head and Neck Surgery. Vol 4, Ear and Cranial Base. St Louis, Mich: Mosby; 2908-2933.

Ash CM, Pinto OF (1991) The TMJ and the middle ear: structural and functional correlates for aural symptoms associated with temporomandibular joint dysfunction. International Journal of Prosthetics 4: 51-57.

Ashmore J, Gale J (2000) The cochlea: a primer. Current Biology 10: R325-327.

Asplund R (2003) Sleepiness and sleep in elderly persons with tinnitus. Archives of Gerontology and Geriatrics 37: 139-145.

Attias J, Weisa G, Almog S (1994) Oral magnesium intake reduces permanent hearing loss induced by noise exposure. American Journal of Otolaryngology 15: 26-32.

Attias J, Shemsh Z, Shoam C, Shahar A, Sohmer H (1990) Efficacy of self-hypnosis for tinnitus relief. Scandinavian Audiology 19: 245-249.

Attias J, Urbach D, Gold S, Shemesh Z (1993a) Auditory event related potentials in chronic tinnitus patients with noise induced hearing loss. Hearing Research 71: 106-113.

Attias J, Shemsh Z, Sohmer H, Gold S, Shoam C, Faraggi D (1993b) Comparison between self-hypnosis, masking and attentiveness for alleviation of chronic tinnitus. Audiology 32: 302-212.

Attias J, Shemsh Z, Bleich A, Solomon Z, Bar-Or G, Alster J et al. (1995) Psychological profile of help-seeking and non-help-seeking tinnitus patients. Scandinavian Audiology 24: 13-18.

Attias J, Furman V, Shemesh Z, Bresloff I (1996a) Impaired brain processing in noise-induced tinnitus patients as measured by auditory and visual event-related potentials. Ear and Hearing 17: 327-333.

Attias J, Pratt H, Bresloff I, Horowitz G, Polyakov A, Shemsh Z (1996b) Detailed analysis of auditory brainstem responses in patients with noise-induced tinnitus. Audiology 35: 259-270.

Axelsson A, Ringdahl A (1989) Tinnitus – a study of its prevalence and characteristics. British Journal of Audiology 23: 53-62.

Axelsson A, Coles R, Erlandsson S, Meikle M, Vernon J (1993) Evaluation of tinnitus treatment: methodological aspects. Journal of Audiological Medicine 2: 141-150.

Axelsson A, Andersson S, Gu L-D (1994) Acupuncture in the management of tinnitus: a placebo controlled study. Audiology 33: 351-360.

Axelsson A, Anari M, Eliasson A (1995) Överkänslighet för Ljud (ÖFL). (Sensitivity to Sound.) Stockholm: Socialstyrelsen.

Ayache D, Earally F, Elbaz P (2003) Characteristics and postoperative course of tinnitus in otosclerosis. Otology and Neurotology 24: 48-51.

Baddeley AD (1986) Working Memory. Oxford: Oxford University Press.

Badia L, Parikh A, Brookes GB (1994) Management of middle ear myoclonus. Journal of Laryngology and Otology 108: 380-382.

Baguley DM (1997) Neurophysiological approach to tinnitus patients (Letter to the Editor). American Journal of Otology 18: 265.

Baguley DM (2002) Mechanisms of tinnitus. British Medical Bulletin 63: 195-212.

Baguley DM, McFerran DJ (1999) Tinnitus in childhood. International Journal of Pediatric Otorhinolaryngology 49: 99-105.

Baguley DM, Andersson G (2002) Comment on Howard. Otology and Neurotology 23: 411-412.

Baguley DM, McFerran DJ (2002) Current perspectives on tinnitus. Archives of Disability in Children 86: 141-143.

Baguley DM, Andersson G (2003) Factor analysis of the Tinnitus Handicap Inventory. American Journal of Audiology 12: 31-34.

Baguley DM, Moffat DA, Hardy DG (1992) What is the effect of translabyrinthine acoustic schwannoma removal upon tinnitus? Journal of Laryngology and Otology 106: 329-331.

Baguley DM, Beynon GJ, Thornton F (1997) A consideration of the effect of ear canal resonance and hearing loss upon white noise generators for tinnitus retraining therapy. Journal of Laryngology and Otology 111: 803-813.

Baguley DM, Stoddart RL, Hodgson CA (2000) Convergent validity of the Tinnitus Handicap Inventory and the Tinnitus Questionnaire. Journal of Laryngology and Otology 114: 840-843.

Baguley DM, Chang P, Moffat DA (2001) Tinnitus in vestibular schwannoma. Seminars in Hearing 22: 77-88.

Baguley DM, Axon P, Winter IM, Moffat DA (2002) The effect of vestibular nerve section upon tinnitus. Clinical Otolaryngology 27: 219-226.

Baguley DM, Davies E, Hazell JWP (2003) A vision for tinnitus research. International Journal of Audiology 42: 2-3.

Banbury SP, Macken WJ, Tremblay S, Jones DM (2001) Auditory distraction and short-term memory: phenomena and practical implications. Human Factors 43: 12-29.

Bárány R (1935) Die beeinflussung des ohrensausens durch intravenös injizierte lokalanästhetica. Acta Otolaryngologica 23: 201-203.

Barlow DH (2001) Clinical Handbook of Psychological Disorders. A Step-by-Step Treatment Manual. New York, NY: Guilford Press.

Barnea G, Attias J, Gold S, Shahar A (1990) Tinnitus with normal hearing sensitivity: extended high-frequency audiometry and auditory-nerve brainstem-evoked responses. Audiology 29: 36-45.

Bartnik G, Fabijanska A, Rogowski M (1999) Our experience in treatment of patients with tinnitus and/or hyperacusis using the habituation method. In: Hazell J (ed.). Proceedings of the Sixth International Tinnitus Seminar. Cambridge: The Tinnitus and Hyperacusis Centre; 415-417.

Bartnik G, Fabijanska A, Rogowski M (2001) Effects of tinnitus retraining therapy (TRT) for patients with tinnitus and subjective hearing loss versus tinnitus only. Scandinavian Audiology 52(suppl): 206-208.

Baskill JL, Bradley PJM, Coles RRA, Graham RL, Grimes S, Handscomb L et al. (1999) Effects of publicity on tinnitus. In: Hazell J (ed.). Proceedings of the Sixth International Tinnitus Seminar. Cambridge: The Tinnitus and Hyperacusis Centre; 229-231.

Basmajian JV (1999) Debonafide effects vs 'Placebo effects'. Proceedings of the Royal College of Physicians Edinburgh 29: 243-244.

Bastien CH, Vallières A, Morin CM (2001) Validation of the Insomnia Severity Index as an outcome measure for insomnia research. Sleep Medicine 2: 297-307.

Bayar N, Boke B, Turan E, Belgin E (2001) Efficacy of amytriptyline in the treatment of subjective tinnitus. Journal of Otolaryngology 30: 300-303.

Beard AW (1965) Results of leucotomy operations for tinnitus. Journal of Psychosomatic Research 9: 29-32.

Beck AT, Ward CH, Mendelson M, Mock J, Erbaugh J (1961) An inventory for measuring depression. Archives of General Psychiatry 4: 561-571.

Bernard PA (1981) Freedom from ototoxicity in aminoglycoside treated neonates: a mistaken notion. Laryngoscope 91: 1985-1994.

Berry JA, Gold SL, Frederick EA, Gray WC, Staecker H (2002) Patient-based outcomes in patients with primary tinnitus undergoing tinnitus retraining therapy. Archives of Otolaryngology – Head and Neck Surgery 128: 1153-1157.

Bhatnagar SC (2002) Neuroscience for the Study of Communicative Disorders. Philadelphia, Pa: Lippincott Williams & Wilkins.

Biggs NDW, Ramsden RT (2002) Gaze-evoked tinnitus following acoustic neuroma resection: a de-afferentation plasticity phenomenon? Clinical Otolaryngology 27: 338-343.

Bjelland I, Dahl AA, Haug TT, Neckelman D (2002) The validity of the hospital anxiety and depression scale. An updated literature review. Journal of Psychosomatic Research 52: 69-77.

Blanchard (1693) Physician's Dictionary. London.

Blanchard EB, Schwartz SP (1988) Clinically significant changes in behavioral medicine. Behavioral Assessment 10: 171-188.

Blaustein MP (1988) Cellular calcium: nervous system. In: Nordin BEC (ed.). Calcium in Human Biology. London: Springer-Verlag; 339-366.

Blayney AW, Phillips MS, Guy AM, Colman BH (1985) A sequential double blind cross-over trial of tocainide hydrochloride in tinnitus. Clinical Otolaryngology 10: 97-101.

Blood AJ, Zatorre RJ, Bermudex P, Evans AC (1999) Emotional responses to pleasant and unpleasant music correlate with activity in paralimbic brain regions. Nature Neuroscience 2: 382-387.

Bornstein SP, Musiek FE (1993) Loudness discomfort level and reliability as a function of instructional set. Scandinavian Audiology 22: 125-131.

Bouscau-Faure F, Keller P, Dauman R (2003) Further validation of the Iowa tinnitus handicap questionnaire. Acta Otolaryngology 123: 227-231.

Brattberg G (1983) An alternative method of treating tinnitus: relaxation-hypnotherapy primarily through the home use of a recorded audio cassette. International Journal of Clinical and Experimental Hypnosis 31: 90-97.

Briner W, Risey J, Guth P, Noris C (1990) Use of the million clinical multiaxial inventory in evaluating patients with severe tinnitus. American Journal of Otolaryngology 11: 334-337.

Broadbent DFCP, Fitzgerald P, Parkes KR (1982) The cognitive failures questionnaire and its correlates. British Journal of Clinical Psychology 21: 1-16.

Brookes GB (1996) Vascular decompression surgery for severe tinnitus. American Journal of Otolology 17: 569-576.

Brookes GB, Maw AR, Coleman MJ (1980) 'Costen's syndrome' – correlation or coincidence: a review of 45 patients with temporomandibular joint dysfunction, otalgia and other aural symptoms. Clinical Otolaryngology 5: 25-36.

Brooks DN, Chalmers P (1991) Training in audiology. British Journal of Audiology 25: 73-75.

Brooks DN (1989) Adult Aural Rehabilitation. London: Chapman & Hall.

Browning GG, Gatehouse S (1992) The prevalence of middle ear disease in the adult British population. Clinical Otolaryngology 17: 317-321.

Budd RJ, Pugh R (1995) The relationship between locus of control, tinnitus severity, and emotional distress in a group of tinnitus sufferers. Journal of Psychosomatic Research 39: 1015-1018.

Budd RJ, Pugh R (1996a) The relationship between coping style, tinnitus severity and emotional distress in a group of tinnitus sufferers. British Journal of Health Psychology 1: 219-229.

Budd RJ, Pugh R (1996b) Tinnitus coping style and its relationship to tinnitus severity and emotional distress. Journal of Psychosomatic Research 40: 327-335.

Burns EM (1984) A comparison of variability among measurements of subjective tinnitus and objective stimuli. Audiology 23: 426–440.

Cacace AT (1999) Delineating tinnitus-related activity in the nervous system: application of functional imaging at the fin de siècle. In: Hazell J (ed.). Proceedings of the Sixth International Tinnitus Seminar. Cambridge: The Tinnitus and Hyperacusis Centre; 39–44.

Cacace AT (2003) Expanding the biological basis of tinnitus: cross-modal origins and the role of neuroplasticity. Hearing Research 175: 112–132.

Cacace AT, Lovely TJ, McFarland DJ, Pames SM, Winter DF (1994) Anomalous cross-modal plasticity following posterior fossa surgery: some speculations on gaze-evoked tinnitus. Hearing Research 81: 22–32.

Cacace AT, Cousins JP, Moonen CTW, van Gelderen P, Miller D, Parnes SM.et al. (1996) *In-vivo* localization of phantom auditory perceptions during functional magnetic resonance imaging of the human brain. In: Reich GE, Vernon JA (eds). Proceedings of the Fifth International Tinnitus Seminar. Portland, Oreg: American Tinnitus Association; 397–401.

Cacace AT, Cousins JC, Pames S, Semenoff D, Holmes T, McFarland DJ et al. (1999a) Cutaneous-evoked tinnitus. I. Phenomenology, psychophysics, and functional imaging. Audiology and Neurootology 4: 247–257.

Cacace AT, Cousins JC, Pames S, McFarland DJ, Semenoff D, Holmes T et al. (1999b) Cutaneous-evoked tinnitus. II. Review of neuroanatomical, physiological, and functional imaging studies. Audiology and Neurootology 4: 258–268.

Cahani M, Paul G, Shahar A (1984) Tinnitus asymmetry. Audiology 23: 127–135.

Campbell K (1993) Tinnitus and vertigo [Letter to the Editor]. Archives of Otolaryngology – Head Neck Surgery 119: 474.

Carlsson SG, Erlandsson SI (1991) Habituation and tinnitus: an experimental study. Journal of Psychosomatic Research 35: 509–514.

Carman JS (1973) Imipramine in hyperacusic depression. American Journal of Psychiatry 130: 937.

Carmen R, Svihovec D (1984) Relaxation – biofeedback in the treatment of tinnitus. American Journal of Otology 5: 376–381.

Carrick DG, Davies WH, Fielder CP, Bihari J (1986) Low-powered ultrasound in the treatment of tinnitus: a pilot study. British Journal of Audiology 20: 153–155.

Catalano PJ, Post KD (1996) Elimination of tinnitus following hearing preservation surgery for acoustic neuromas. American Journal of Otology 17: 443–445

Cawthorne T, Hewlett AB (1954) Ménière's disease. Proceedings of the Royal Society of Medicine 47: 663–670.

Chan SWY, Reade PC (1994) Tinnitus and temporomandibular pain–dysfunction disorder. Clinical Otolaryngology 19: 370–380.

Chen G, Jastreboff PJ (1995) Salicylate induced abnormal activity in the inferior colliculus of rats. Hearing Research 82: 158–178.

Chen K, Chang H, Zhang J, Kaltenbach JA, Godfrey DA (1999) Altered spontaneous activity in rat dorsal cochlea nucleus following loud tone exposure. In: Hazell J (ed.). Proceedings of the Sixth International Tinnitus Seminar. Cambridge: The Tinnitus and Hyperacusis Centre; 212–217.

Chiossoine-Kerdel JA, Baguley DM, Stoddart RL, Moffat DA (2000) An investigation of the audiological handicap associated with unilateral sudden sensorineural hearing loss. American Journal of Otology 21: 645–651.

Chouard CH, Meyer B, Maridat D (1981) Transcutaneous electrotherapy for severe tinnitus. Acta Otolaryngology 91: 415–422.

Clark WW, Kim DO, Zurek PM, Bohne BA (1984) Spontaneous otoacoustic emissions in chinchilla ear canals: correlation with histopathology and suppression by external tones. Hearing Research 16: 299-314.

Cohen J (1988) Statistical Power Analysis for the Behavioral Sciences. Hillsdale, NJ: Lawrence Erlbaum Associates.

Colding-Jørgensen E, Lauritzen M, Johnsen NJ, Mikkelsen KB, Særmark K (1992) On the evidence of auditory evoked magnetic fields as an objective measure of tinnitus. Electroencephalography and Clinical Neurophysiology 83: 322-327.

Coles R, Bradley P, Donaldson I, Dingle A (1991) A trial of tinnitus therapy with ear-canal magnets. Clinical Otolaryngology 16: 371-372.

Coles RRA (1984) Epidemiology of tinnitus: (2) Demographics and clinical features. Journal of Laryngology and Otology 9 (Suppl.): 195-202.

Coles RRA (1987) Tinnitus and its management. In: Stephens D (ed.). Adult Audiology. Scott Brown's Otolaryngology (fifth edition). London: Butterworths; 368-414.

Coles RRA (1992) A survey of tinnitus management in national health service hospitals. Clinical Otolaryngology 17: 313-316.

Coles RRA, Hallam RS (1987) Tinnitus and its management. British Medical Bulletin 43: 983-998.

Coles RRA, Thompson AC, O'Donoghue GM (1992) Intra-tympanic injections in the treatment of tinnitus. Clinical Otolaryngology 17: 240-242.

Collet L, Moussu MF, Disant F, Ahami T, Morgon A (1990) Minnesota multiphasic personality inventory in tinnitus disorders. Audiology 29: 101-106.

Committee on Hearing and Equilibrium (1995) Guidelines for the diagnosis and evaluation of therapy in Ménière's disease. Otolaryngology, Head and Neck Surgery 113: 181-185.

Cooper JC (1994) Health and nutrition examination survey of 1971-75: part II. Tinnitus, subjective hearing loss, and well-being, Journal of the American Academy of Audiology 5: 37-43.

Cortopassi G, Hutchin T (1994) A molecular and cellular hypothesis for aminoglycoside induced deafness. Hearing Research 78: 27-30.

Costen JB (1934) A syndrome of ear and sinus symptoms dependent upon disturbed function of the temporomandibular joint. Annals of Otology, Rhinology and Laryngology 43: 1-15.

Coyle PK, Schutzer SE (2002) Neurological aspects of Lyme disease. Medical Clinics of North America 86: 261-284.

Dauman R (2000) Electrical stimulation for tinnitus suppression. In Tyler RS (Ed.) Tinnitus Handbook. San Diego, Calif: Singular, Thomson Learning; 377-398.

Dauman R, Tyler RS (1992) Some considerations on the classification of tinnitus. In: Aran J-M, Dauman R (eds). Tinnitus '91. Proceedings of the Fourth International Tinnitus Seminar. Amsterdam: Kugler Publications; 225-229.

Dauman R, Tyler RS (1993) Tinnitus suppression in cochlear implant users. Advances in Otorhinolaryngology 48: 168-173.

Davies S, McKenna L, Hallam RS (1995) Relaxation and cognitive therapy: a controlled trial in chronic tinnitus. Psychology and Health 10: 129-143.

Davies WE, Knox E, Donaldson K (1994). The usefulness of nipodipine, an L-calcium channel antagonist, in the treatment of tinnitus. British Journal of Audiology 28: 125-129.

Davis A (1995) Hearing in Adults. London: Whurr Publishers.

Davis AC (1989) The prevalence of hearing impairment and reported hearing disability among adults in Great Britain. International Journal of Epidemiology 18: 911-917.

Davis A, El Rafaie A (2000) Epidemiology of tinnitus. In: Tyler RS (ed.). Tinnitus Handbook. San Diego, Calif: Singular, Thomson Learning; 1-23.

Davis M, Astrachan DI, Kass E (1980) Excitatory and inhibitory effects of serotonin on sensorimotor reactivity measured with acoustic startle. Science 209: 521-523.

DeBartolo HM (1989) Zinc and diet for tinnitus. American Journal of Otology 10: 256.

De Houwer J, Thomas S, Baeyens F (2001) Associative learning of likes and dislikes: a review of 25 years of research on human evaluative conditioning. Psychological Bulletin 127: 853-869.

den Hartig J, Hilders CGJM, Schoemaker RC, Hulsohof JH, Cohen AF, Vermeij P (1993) Tinnitus suppression by intravenous lidocaine in relation to its plasma concentration. Clinical Pharmacology and Therapeutics 54: 415-420.

Denk D, Heinzl H, Franz P, Ehrenberger K (1997). Caroverine in tinnitus treatment. Acta Otolaryngologica 117: 825-830.

Dineen R, Doyle J, Bench J. (1997a) Audiological and psychological characteristics of a group of tinnitus sufferers, prior to tinnitus management training. British Journal of Audiology 31: 27-38.

Dineen R, Doyle J, Bench J (1997b) Managing tinnitus: a comparison of different approaches to tinnitus management training. British Journal of Audiology 31: 331-344.

Dobie RA (1999) A review of randomized clinical trials of tinnitus. Laryngoscope 109: 1202-1211.

Dobie RA (2002) Randomised clinical trials for tinnitus: not the last word? In: Patuzzi RL (ed.). Proceedings of the Seventh International Tinnitus Seminar. Freemantle: University of Western Australia; 3-6.

Dobie RA, Hoberg KE, Rees TS (1986) Electrical tinnitus suppression: a double-blind crossover study. Otolaryngology, Head and Neck Surgery 95: 319-323.

Douek E (1981) Classification of tinnitus. In: Evered D, Lawrenson G (eds). Tinnitus, Ciba Foundation symposium 85. London: Pitman Books; 4-15.

Douek E, Reid J (1968) The diagnostic value of tinnitus pitch. Journal of Laryngology and Otology 82: 1039-1042.

Donaldson I (1981) Tegretol: a double blind trial in tinnitus. Journal of Laryngology and Otology 95: 947-951.

Drukier GS (1989) The prevalence and characteristics of tinnitus with profound sensorineural hearing impairment. American Annals of the Deaf 134: 260-264.

Duckert LG, Rees TS (1984) Placebo effect in tinnitus management. Otolaryngology, Head and Neck Surgery 92: 697-699.

DuVerney JG (1683) Traité de l'Organe de l'Ouie. Paris: Michallet.

Drew S, Davies E (2001) Effectiveness of Ginkgo Biloba in treating tinnitus: double blind, placebo controlled trial. British Medical Journal 322: 1-6.

Egger M, Davey Smith G (1997) Meta-analysis: potentials and promise. British Medical Journal 315: 1371-1374.

Eggermont JJ (1990) On the pathophysiology of tinnitus; a review and a peripheral model. Hearing Research 48: 111-124.

Eggermont JJ (2000) Physiological mechanisms and neural models, In: Tyler RS (ed.). Tinnitus Handbook. San Diego, Calif: Singular, Thomson Learning; 85-122.

Eisenberg DM, Davis RB, Ettner SL, Appel S, Wilkey S, Van Rompay M et al. (1998) Trends in alternative medicine use in the United States, 1990-1997: results of a follow-up national survey. Journal of the American Medical Association 280: 1569-1575.

El Rafaie A, Davis A, Baskill JL, Lovell E, Taylor A, Spencer H et al. (1999) Quality of family life of people who report tinnitus. In: Hazell J (ed.). Proceedings of the Sixth International Tinnitus Seminar. Cambridge: The Tinnitus and Hyperacusis Centre; 45-50.

Erlandsson S (1990) Tinnitus: tolerance or threat? Psychological and psychophysiological perspectives. Doctoral thesis. University of Göteborg: Department of Psychology.

Erlandsson S (2000) Psychological profile of tinnitus patients. In: Tyler RS (ed.). Tinnitus Handbook. San Diego, Calif: Singular, Thomson Learning; 25-57.

Erlandsson S, Ringdahl A, Hutchins T, Carlsson SG (1987) Treatment of tinnitus: a controlled comparison of masking and placebo. British Journal of Audiology 21: 37-44.

Erlandsson S, Rubenstein B, Carlsson SG (1991) Tinnitus: evaluation of biofeedback and stomatognatic treatment. British Journal of Audiology 25: 151-161.

Erlandsson SI, Eriksson-Mangold M, Wiberg A (1996) Ménière's disease: trauma, distress and adaption studied through focus interview analyses. Scandinavian Audiology 25 (Suppl. 43): 45-56.

Erlandsson SI, Hallberg LRM, Axelsson A (1992) Psychological and audiological correlates of perceived tinnitus severity. Audiology 31: 168-179.

Ernst E (2002) The risk-benefit profile of commonly used herbal therapies: ginkgo, St John's wort, gingseng, echinacea, saw palmetto, and kava. Annals of Internal Medicine 136: 42-53.

Ernst E, Stevinson C (1999) Ginkgo biloba for tinnitus: a review. Clinical Otolaryngology 24: 164-167.

Evans D (2003) Placebo. The Belief Effect. London: Harper Collins.

Evans EF, Wilson JP, Borerwe TA (1981) Animal models of tinnitus. In: Evered D, Lawrenson G (eds). Tinnitus. Ciba Foundation Symposium 85. London: Pitman Books; 108-138.

Eysenck H, Eysenck S (1975) Manual of the Eysenck Personality Questionnaire. London: Hodder & Stoughton.

Fabijanska A, Rogowski M, Bartnik G, Skarzynski H (1999) Epidemiology of tinnitus and hyperacusis in Poland. In: Hazell J (ed.). Proceedings of the Sixth International Tinnitus Seminar. Cambridge: The Tinnitus and Hyperacusis Centre; 569-571.

Feldmann H (1971) Homolateral and contralateral masking of tinnitus by noise-bands and pure tones. Audiology 10: 138-144.

Feldmann H (1997) A history of tinnitus research. In: Shulman A (ed.). Tinnitus: Diagnosis/Treatment. San Diego, Calif: Singular; 3-40.

Filipo R, Barbara M, Cordier A, Mafera B, Romeo R, Attanasio G. et al. (1997) Osmotic drugs in the treatment of cochlear disorders: a clinical and experimental study. Acta Otolaryngology 117: 229-231.

First MB, Gibbon M, Spitzer RL, Williams JBW (1997) Structured Clinical Interview for DSM-IV Axis I Disorders (SCID-I). Washington, DC: American Psychiatric Press.

Fishman RA (1980) Benign intracranial hypertension. Cerebrospinal Fluid in Disease of the Nervous System. Philadelphia, Pa: WB Saunders; 128-139.

FitzGerald M, Folan-Curran J (2002) Clinical Neuroanatomy and Related Neuroscience. Edinburgh: WB Saunders.

Flor H, Fydrich T, Turk DC (1992) Efficacy of multidisciplinary treatment centers: a meta-analytic review. Pain 49: 221-230.

Folmer RL (2002) Long-term reductions in tinnitus severity. BMC Ear, Nose and Throat Disorders 2. (www.biomedcentral.com/1472-6815/2/3)

Folmer RL, Greist SE (2000) Tinnitus and insomnia. American Journal of Otolaryngology 21: 287-293.

Folmer RL, Griest SE, Bonaduce A, Edlefsen LL (2002) Use of serotonin reuptake inhibitors (SSRIs) by patients with chronic tinnitus. In: Patuzzi RL (ed.). Proceedings of the Seventh International Tinnitus Seminar. Freemantle: University of Western Australia; 81- 85.

Fowler EP (1936) A method for the early detection of otosclerosis. Archives of Otolaryngology 24: 731-741.

Fowler EP (1941) Tinnitus aurium in the light of recent research. Annals of Otology 50: 139-158.

Fowler EP (1942) The 'illusion of loudness' of tinnitus - its etiology and treatment. Laryngoscope 52: 275-285.

Fowler EP (1944) Head noises in normal and disordered ears. Significance, measurement, differentiation and treatment. Archives of Otolaryngology 39: 498-503.

Fowler EP (1948) The emotional factor in tinnitus aurium. Laryngoscope 58: 145-154.

Fowler EP (1953) Intravenous procaine in the treatment of Ménière's disease. Annals of Otology, Rhinology and Laryngology 62: 1186-1200.

Fowler EP, Fowler EPJ (1955) Somatopsychic and psychosomatic factors in tinnitus, deafness and vertigo. Annals of Otology, Rhinology, and Laryngology 64: 29-37.

Furugård S, Hedin P-J, Eggertz A, Laurent C (1998) Akupunktur värt att pröva vid svår tinnitus. Läkartidningen 95: 1922-1928.

Frankenburg FR, Hegarty JD (1994) Tinnitus, psychosis and suicide. Archives of Internal Medicine 154: 2371-2372.

Fredrikson M, Furmark T (2003) Amygdaloid regional cerebral blood flow and subjective fear during symptom provocation in anxiety disorders. Annals of the New York Academy of Science 985: 341-347.

Fritsch MH, Wynne MK, Matt BH, Smith WL, Smith CM (2001) Objective tinnitus in children. Otology and Neurotology 22: 644-649.

Gabriels P (1993) Hyperacusis - can we help? Australian Journal of Audiology 15: 1-4.

Gabriels P (1995) Children with tinnitus. In: Reich G, Vernon J (eds). Proceedings of the Fifth International Tinnitus Seminar. Portland, Oreg: The American Tinnitus Association: 270-274.

Gardner A, Pagani M, Jacobsson H, Lindberg G, Larsson SA, Wägner A et al. (2002) Differences in resting state regional cerebral blood flow assessed with 99mTc-HMPAO SPECT and brain atlas matching between depressed patients with or without tinnitus, Nuclear Medicine Communications 23: 429-439.

Gelb H, Bernstein I (1983) Clinical evaluation of two hundred patients with temporomandibular joint syndrome. Journal of Prosthetic Dentistry 49: 234-243.

George RN, Kemp S (1991) A survey of New Zealanders with tinnitus. British Journal of Audiology 25: 331-336.

Gerken GM (1996) Central tinnitus and lateral inhibition: an auditory brainstem model. Hearing Research 97: 75-83.

Gerken GM, Hesse PS, Wiorkowski JJ (2001) Auditory evoked responses in control subjects and in patients with problem-tinnitus. Hearing Research 157: 52-64.

Gersdorff M, Nouwen J, Gilain C, Decat M, Betsch C (2000) Tinnitus and otosclerosis. European Archives of Otorhinolaryngology 257: 314-316.

Gersdorff M, Robinillard T, Steinm F, Declaye X, Vanderbemden S (1987) A clinical correlation between hypozincemia and tinnitus. Archives of Otorhinolaryngology 244: 190-193.

Ghatan P, Ingvar DH, Stone-Elander S, Ingvar M (1996) Serial seven, an arithmetical test of working memory and attention: a PET study. Neuroimage 3: S179.

Ghatan PH, Hsieh JC, Petersson KM, Stone-Elander S, Ingvar M (1998) Coexistence of attention-based facilitation and inhibition in the human cortex. Neuroimage 7: 23-29.

Gibson R (1973) Paget's disease of the temporal bone. Acta Otolaryngologica 87: 299-301.

Gibson WP, Arenberg IK (1997) Pathophysiologic theories in the etiology of Ménière's disease. Otolaryngologic Clinics of North America 30: 961-967.

Giraud AL, Chéry-Croze S, Fischer G, Fischer C, Vighetto A, Grégoire M-C et al. (1999) A selective imaging of tinnitus. NeuroReport 10: 1-5.

Goebel G, Hiller W (1999) Quality management in the therapy of chronic tinnitus. In: Hazell J (Ed.). Proceedings of the Sixth International Tinnitus Seminar. Cambridge: The Tinnitus and Hyperacusis Centre; 357-363.

Gold S, Formby C, Frederick EA, Suter C (2002) Shifts in loudness discomfort level in tinnitus patients with and without hyperacusis. In: Patuzzi R (ed.). Proceedings of the Seventh International Tinnitus Seminar. Freemantle: University of Western Australia; 170-172.

Gold T (1948) Hearing.II. The physical basis of the action of the cochlea. Proceedings of the Royal Society of Edinburgh (Biological Sciences) 135: 492-498.

Goldberg D (1978) Manual of the General Health Questionnaire. Slough: National Foundation for Educational Research.

Goodey RJ (1981) Drugs in the treatment of tinnitus. In: Evered D, Lawrenson G (eds). Tinnitus, Ciba Foundation Symposium 85. London: Pitman Books; 263-278.

Goodwin PE, Johnson RM (1980a) The loudness of tinnitus. Acta Otolaryngology 90: 353-359.

Goodwin PE, Johnson RM (1980b) A comparison of reaction times to tinnitus and nontinnitus frequencies. Ear and Hearing 1: 148-155.

Graham JM (1981) In: Evered D, Lawrenson G (eds) Tinnitus, Ciba Foundation Symposium 85. London: Pitman Books; 172-192.

Graham JM (1987) Tinnitus in hearing impaired children. In: Hazell JWP (ed.) Tinnitus. London: Churchill Livingstone; 131-143.

Graham JT, Newby HA (1962) Acoustical characteristics of tinnitus. Archives of Otolaryngology 75: 162-167.

Granqvist P, Lantto S, Ortiz L, Andersson G (2001) Adult attachment, perceived family support, and problems experienced by tinnitus patients. Psychology and Health 16: 357-366.

Green JD, Blum DJ, Harner SG (1991) Longitudinal follow up of patients with Ménière's disease. Otolaryngology, Head, and Neck Surgery 104: 783-788.

Groves PM, Thompson RF (1970) Habituation: a dual process theory. Psychological Review 77: 419-450.

Gu L-D, Axelsson A (1996) Acupuncture for tinnitus: a review from five years of clinical investigations. In: Reich GE, Vernon JA (eds). Proceedings of the Fifth International Tinnitus Seminar 1995. Portland, Oreg: American Tinnitus Association; 84-89.

Guitton MJ, Caston J, Ruel J, Johnson RM, Pujol R, Puel JL (2003) Salicylate induces tinnitus through activation of cochlear NMDA receptors. Journal of Neuroscience 23: 3944-3952.

Gulya AJ, Schuknecht HF (1995) Anatomy of the Temporal Bone with Surgical Implications. New York, NY: Parthenon.

Haerkötter C, Hiller W (2002) Combining elements of tinnitus retraining therapy (TRT) and cognitive-behavioral therapy: does it work? In: Patuzzi R (ed.). Proceedings of the Seventh International Tinnitus Seminar. Freemantle: University of Western Australia; 7.

Halford JBS, Anderson SD (1991a) Tinnitus severity measured by a subjective scale, audiometry and clinical judgement. Journal of Laryngology and Otology 105: 89-93.

Halford JBS, Anderson SD (1991b) Anxiety and depression in tinnitus sufferers. Journal of Psychosomatic Research 35: 383-390.

Hall JW III (2000) Handbook of Otoacoustic Emissions. San Diego, Calif: Singular.

Hallam R, McKenna L, Shurlock L (2004) Tinnitus impairs cognitive efficiency. International Journal of Audiology.

Hallam RS (1987) Psychological approaches to the evaluation and management of tinnitus distress. In: Hazell J (ed.). Tinnitus. London: Churchill-Livingstone; 156-175.

Hallam RS (1989) Living with Tinnitus: Dealing With the Ringing in Your Ears. Wellingborough: Thorsons.

Hallam RS (1996a) Manual of the Tinnitus Questionnaire. London: The Psychological Corporation/Brace & Co.

Hallam RS (1996b) Correlates of sleep disturbances in chronic distressing tinnitus. Scandinavian Audiology 25: 263-266.

Hallam RS, Rachman S, Hinchcliffe R (1984) Psychological aspects of tinnitus. In: Rachman S (ed.). Contributions to Medical Psychology, Vol. 3. Oxford: Pergamon Press; 31-53

Hallam RS, Jakes SC, Hinchcliffe R (1988) Cognitive variables in tinnitus annoyance. British Journal of Clinical Psychology 27: 213-222.

Hallam RS, McKenna L, Shurlock L (2004) Tinnitus impairs cognitive function. International Journal of Audiology 43: 1-9.

Hallberg LR-M, Erlandsson SI, Carlsson SG (1992) Coping strategies used by middle-aged males with noise-induced hearing loss, with and without tinnitus. Psychology and Health 7: 273-288.

Hallberg LR-M, Erlandsson SI (1993) Tinnitus characteristics in tinnitus complainers and noncomplainers. British Journal of Audiology 27: 19-27.

Hallpike CS, Cairns H (1938) Observations on the pathology of Ménière's syndrome. Journal of Laryngology and Otology 53: 625.

Hansen PE, Hansen JH, Bentzen O (1982) Acupuncture treatment of chronic unilateral tinnitus – a double-blind cross-over trial. Clinical Otolaryngology 7: 325-329.

Haralambous G, Wilson PH, Platt-Hepworth S, Tonkin JP, Hensley VR, Kavanagh D (1987) EMG biofeedback in the treatment of tinnitus: an experimental evaluation. Behaviour Research and Therapy 25: 49-55.

Harrison RV, Nagasawa A, Smith DW, Stanton S, Stanton JMR (1991) Reorganisation of auditory cortex after neonatal high frequency coclear hearing loss. Hearing Research 54: 11-19.

Harrop-Griffiths J, Katon W, Dobie R, Sakai C, Russo J (1987) Chronic tinnitus: association with psychiatric diagnoses. Journal of Psychosomatic Research 31: 613-621.

Hathaway SR, McKinley JC (1940) A multiphasic personality schedule (Minnesota). I. Construction of the schedule. Journal of Psychology 10: 249-254.

Hauri PJ (1993) Consulting about insomnia: a method and some preliminary data. Sleep 16: 344-350.

Hazell J (1991) Tinnitus and disability in ageing. Acta Oto-Laryngologica 476 (Suppl.): 202-208.

Hazell (1995).

Hazell JWP (1987) A cochlear model for tinnitus. In: Feldmann H (ed.). Proceedings of the Third International Tinnitus Seminar. Karlsruhe: Harsch Verlag; 121-128.

Hazell JWP (1996) Support for a neurophysiological model of tinnitus. In: Reich GE, Vernon JA (eds). Proceedings of the Fifth International Tinnitus Seminar 1995. Portland, Oreg: American Tinnitus Association; 51-57.

Hazell JWP, Jastreboff PJ (1990) Tinnitus I: Auditory mechanisms: a model for tinnitus and hearing impairment. Journal of Otolaryngology 19: 1-5.

Hazell JWP, Sheldrake JB (1992) Hyperacusis and tinnitus. In: Aran J-M, Dauman R (eds). Tinnitus '91. Proceedings of the Fourth International Tinnitus Seminar. Amsterdam: Kugler Publications; 245-248.

Hazell JWP, Sheldrake JB, Graham RL (2002) Decreased sound tolerance: predisposing factors, triggers and outcomes after TRT. In: Patuzzi R (ed.). Proceedings of the Seventh International Tinnitus Seminar. Freemantle: University of Western Australia; 255-261.

Hazell JWP, Wood SM, Cooper HR, Stephens SDG, Corcoran AL, Coles RRA et al. (1985) A clinical study of tinnitus maskers. British Journal of Audiology 19: 65-146.

Heimer L (1995) The Human Brain and Spinal Cord: Functional Neuroanatomy and Dissection Guide (second edition). New York, NY: Springer-Verlag.

Heitzmann T, Rubio L, Cardenas MR, Zofio E (1999) The importance of continuity in TRT patients: results at 18 months. In: Hazell J (ed.). Proceedings of the Sixth International Tinnitus Seminar. Cambridge: The Tinnitus and Hyperacusis Centre; 509–511.

Heller MF, Bergman M (1953) Tinnitus aurium in normally hearing persons. Annals of Otology, Rhinology and Laryngology 62: 73–83.

Helm J (1981) Tympanoplastik und ohrgerauscke. Laryngology, Rhinology and Otology 60: 99–100.

Henry J, Wilson P (2001) Psychological Management of Chronic Tinnitus. A Cognitive-behavioral Approach. Boston, Mass: Allyn & Bacon.

Henry JA, Meikle MB (1999) Pulsed versus continous tones for evaluating the loudness of tinnitus. Journal of the American Academy of Audiology 10: 261–272.

Henry JA, Meikle MB (2000) Psychoacoustic measures of tinnitus. Journal of the American Academy of Audiology 11: 138–155.

Henry JA, Flick CL, Gilbert A, Ellingson RM, Fausti SA (1999) Reliability of tinnitus loudness matches under procedural variation. Journal of the American Academy of Audiology 10: 502–520.

Henry JA, Schechter MA, Nagler SM, Fausti SA (2002a) Comparison of tinnitus masking and tinnitus retraining therapy. Journal of the American Academy of Audiology 13: 559–581.

Henry JA, Jastreboff MM, Jastreboff PJ, Schechter MA, Fausti SA (2002b) Assessment of patients for treatment with tinnitus retraining therapy. Journal of the American Academy of Audiology 13: 523–544.

Henry JL, Wilson PH (1995) Coping with tinnitus: two studies of psychological and audiological characteristics of patients with high and low tinnitus-related distress. International Tinnitus Journal 1: 85–92.

Henry JL, Wilson PH (1998) An evaluation of two types of cognitive intervention in the management of chronic tinnitus. Scandinavian Journal of Behaviour Therapy 27: 156–166.

Herraiz C, Hernandez FJ, Machado A, De Lucas P, Tapia MM (1999) Tinnitus retraining therapy: our experience. In: Hazell J (ed.). Proceedings of the Sixth International Tinnitus Seminar. Cambridge: The Tinnitus and Hyperacusis Centre, Cambridge; 483–484.

Herraiz C, Hernandez Calvin J, Plaza G, Tapia M, de los Santos G (2001) Evaluacion de la incapacidad en los pacientes con acufenos. Acta Otorrinolaringologica Espanol 52: 534–538.

Hiller W, Goebel G (1992a) A psychometric study of complaints in chronic tinnitus. Journal of Psychosomatic Research 36: 337–348.

Hiller W, Goebel G (1992b) Psychiatric disorders and their degree of severity in patients with severe tinnitus and pain syndromes. In: Aran J-M, Dauman R (eds). Tinnitus '91. Proceedings of the Fourth International Tinnitus Seminar. Amsterdam: Kugler Publications; 441–444.

Hiller W, Goebel G (1999) Assessing audiological, pathophysiological, and psychological variables in chronic tinnitus: a study of reliability and search for prognostic factors. International Journal of Behavioral Medicine 6: 312–330.

Hinchcliffe R (1961) Prevalence of the commoner ear, nose, and throat conditions in the adult rural population of Great Britain. British Journal of Preventive and Social Medicine 15: 128–140.

Hinchcliffe R, Chambers C (1983) Loudness of tinnitus: an approach to measurement. Advances in Oto-Rhino-Laryngology 29: 163–173.

Hinchcliffe R, King PF (1992) Medicolegal aspects of tinnitus. 1: Medicolegal position and current state of knowledge. Journal of Audiological Medicine 1: 38-58.

Hoke M, Feldmann H, Pantev C, Lütkenhöner B, Lehnertz K (1989) Objective evidence of tinnitus in auditory evoked magnetic fields. Hearing Research 37: 281-286.

Hoke ES, Mühlnickel W, Ross B, Hoke M (1998) Tinnitus and event-related activity of the auditory cortex. Audiology and Neuro-Otology 3: 300-331.

Holgers K-M (2003) Tinnitus in 7-year-old children. European Journal of Pediatrics 162: 276-278.

Holgers K-M, Axelsson A, Pringle I (1994) Ginkgo biloba for the treatment of tinnitus. Audiology 33: 85-92.

Holgers K-M, Barrenäs M-L (2003) The pathophysiology and assessment of tinnitus. In: Luxon L, Furman JM, Martini A, Stephens D (eds). Textbook of Audiological Medicine. Clinical Aspects of Hearing and Balance. London: Martin Dunitz; 555-569.

Holgers K-M, Erlandsson SI, Barrenäs M-L (2000) Predictive factors for the severity of tinnitus. Audiology 39: 284-291.

Holley MC (1996) Outer hair cell motility. In: Dallos P, Popper AN, Fay RR (eds). The Cochlea. New York, NY: Springer; 386-434.

Horvath T (1980) Arousal and anxiety. In: Burrows GD, Davis B (eds). Handbook of Studies in Anxiety. North Holland: Elsevier.

House J (1981) Panel on tinnitus control: management of the tinnitus patient. Annals of Otorynolaryngology 90: 597-601.

House JW (1978) Treatment of severe tinnitus with biofeedback training. Laryngoscope 88: 406-412.

House JW, Miller L, House PR (1977) Severe tinnitus: treatment with biofeedback training (results in 41 cases). Transactions of the American Academy of Ophthalmology and Otology 84: 697-703.

Howard ML (2001) Myths in neurotology, revisited: smoke and mirrors in tinnitus therapy. Otology and Neurotology 22: 711-714.

Hughes GB (1998) Sudden hearing loss. In: Gates GA (ed.). Current Therapy in Otolaryngology – Head and Neck Surgery (sixth edition). St Louis, Mich: Mosby; 41-44.

Hurley LM, Thompson AM, Pollack GD (2002) Serotonin in the inferior colliculus. Hearing Research 168: 1-11.

Hypericum Depression Trial Study Group (2002) Effect of hypericum peforatum (St John's wort) in major depressive disorder. Journal of the American Medical Association 287: 1807-1814.

Ikner CL, Hassen AH (1990) The effect of tinnitus on ABR latencies. Ear and Hearing 11: 16-20.

Ince LP, Greene RY, Alba A, Zaretsky HH (1987) A matching-to-sample feedback technique for training self-control of tinnitus. Health Psychology 6: 173-182.

Ireland CE, Wilson PH, Tonkin JP, Platt-Hepworth S (1985) An evaluation of relaxation training in the treatment of tinnitus. Behaviour Research and Therapy 23: 423-430.

Iversen S, Kupfermann I, Kandel ER (2000) Emotional states and feelings. In: Kandel ER, Schwartz JH, Jessel TM (eds). Principles of Neural Science. New York, NY: McGraw-Hill; 982-996.

Jacobson G, McCaslin D (2001) A search for evidence of a direct relationship between tinnitus and suicide. Journal of the American Acadamy of Audiology 12: 493-496.

Jacobson GP, Ahmad BK, Moran J, Newman CW, Tepley N, Wharton J (1991) Auditory evoked cortical magnetic field (M100-M200) measurements in tinnitus and normal groups. Hearing Research 56: 44-52.

Jacobson GP, Calder JA, Newman CW, Peterson EL, Wharton JA, Ahmad BK (1996) Electrophysiological indices of selective auditory attention in subjects with and without tinnitus. Hearing Research 97: 66-74.

Jakes SC, Hallam RS, Chambers C, Hinchcliffe R (1985) A factor analytical study of tinnitus complaint behaviour. Audiology 24: 195-206.

Jakes SC, Hallam RS, McKenna L, Hinchcliffe R (1992) Group therapy for medical patients: an application to tinnitus. Cognitive Therapy and Research 16: 67-82.

Jannetta PJ (1998) Microvascular decompression surgery for tinnitus. In: Vernon JA (ed.). Tinnitus. Treatment and Relief. Boston, Mass: Allyn & Bacon; 218-222.

Jastreboff MM (1999) Controversies between cognitive therapies and TRT counselling. In: Hazell J (ed.). Proceedings of the Sixth International Tinnitus Seminar. Cambridge: The Tinnitus and Hyperacusis Centre; 288-291.

Jastreboff PJ (1990) Phantom auditory perception (tinnitus): mechanisms of generation and perception. Neuroscience Research 8: 221-254.

Jastreboff PJ (1995) Tinnitus as a phantom perception: theories and clinical implications. In: Vernon JA, Møller AR. Mechanisms of Tinnitus. Boston, Mass: Allyn & Bacon; 73-94.

Jastreboff PJ (1998) Tinnitus. In: Gates G (ed.) Current Therapy in Otorhinolaryngology – Head and Neck Surgery. St Lois, MO: Mosby; 90-95.

Jastreboff PJ (1999) The neurophysiological model of tinnitus and hyperacusis. In: Hazell J (ed.). Proceedings of the Sixth International Tinnitus Seminar. Cambridge: The Tinnitus and Hyperacusis Centre; 32-38.

Jastreboff PJ (2000) Tinnitus habituation therapy (THT) and tinnitus retraining therapy (TRT). In: Tyler RS (ed.). Tinnitus Handbook. San Diego, Calif: Singular, Thomson Learning; 357-376.

Jastreboff PJ, Sasaki CT (1986) Salicylate induced changes in spontaneous activity of single units in the inferior colliculus of the guinea pig. Journal of the Acoustic Society of America 50: 1384-1391.

Jastreboff PJ, Hazell JWP (1993) A neurophysiological approach to tinnitus: clinical implications. British Journal of Audiology 27: 7-17.

Jastreboff PJ, Sasaki CT (1994) An animal model of tinnitus: a decade of development. American Journal of Otology 15: 19-27.

Jastreboff PJ, Jastreboff MM (2000) Tinnitus retraining therapy (TRT) as a method for treatment of tinnitus and hyperacusis patients. Journal of the American Academy of Audiology 11: 162-177.

Jastreboff PJ, Jastreboff MM (2001) Tinnitus retraining therapy. Seminars in Hearing 22: 51-63.

Jastreboff PJ, Jastreboff MM (2003) Tinnitus retraining treatment for patients with tinnitus and decreased sound tolerance. Otolaryngologic Clinics of North America 36: 321-336.

Jastreboff PJ, Brennan JF, Coleman JK, Sasaki CT (1988) Phantom auditory sensation in rats: an animal model for tinnitus. Behavioral Neuroscience 102: 811-822.

Jastreboff PJ, Brennan JF, Sasaki CT (1991) Quinine-induced tinnitus in rats. Archives of Otolaryngology, Head, and Neck Surgery 117: 1162-1166.

Jastreboff PJ, Hazell JWP, Graham RL (1994) Neurophysiological model of tinnitus: dependence of the minimal masking level on treatment outcome. Hearing Research 80: 216-232.

Jastreboff PJ, Gray WC, Gold SL (1996) Neurophysiological approach to tinnitus patients. American Journal of Otology 17: 236-240.

Jastreboff PJ, Hazell J (2004) Tinnitus retraining therapy: Implementing the neurophysiological mode. Cambridge: Cambridge University Press.

Jayarajan V, Coles R (1993). Treatment of tinnitus with frusemide. Journal of Audiological Medicine 2: 114-119.

Jensen I, Nygren Å, Gamberale F, Goldie I, Westerholm P, Jonsson E (1995) The role of the psychologist in multidisciplinary treatments for chronic neck and shoulder pain: a controlled cost-effectiveness study. Scandinavian Journal of Rehabilitation Medicine 27: 19-26.

Job RFS (1996) The influence of subjective reactions to noise on health effects of the noise. Environmental International 22: 93-104.

Johansson MSK, Arlinger SD (2003) Prevalence of hearing impairments in a population in Sweden. International Journal of Audiology 42: 18-28.

Johnson RM, Brummett R, Schleuning A (1993) Use of alprazolam for relief of tinnitus. A double-blind study. Archives of Otolaryngology, Head, and Neck Surgery 119: 842-845.

Johnsrude IS, Giraud AL, Frackowiak RSJ (2002) Functional imaging of the auditory system: the use of positron emission tomography. Audiology and Neuro-Otology 7: 251-276.

Johnston M, Walker M (1996) Suicide in the elderly. Recognizing the signs. General Hospital Psychiatry 18: 257-260.

Jones DM, Macken WJ (1993) Irrelevant tones produce an irrelevant speech effect. Journal of Experimental Psychology: Learning, Memory, and Cognition 19: 369-381.

Jones IH, Knudsen VO (1928) Certain aspects of tinnitus, particularly treatment. Laryngoscope 38: 597-611.

Josephson EM (1931) A method of measurement of tinnitus. Archives of Otolaryngology 14: 282-283.

Jung TTK, Rhee CK, Lee CS, Park YS, Choi DC (1993) Ototoxicity of salicylate, nonsteroidal anti-inflammatory drugs, and quinine. Otolaryngolic Clinics of North America 26: 791-810.

Jung TTK, Kim JPS, Bumme J, Davamony D, Duncan J, Fletcher WH (1997) Effect of leukotrine inhibitor on salicylate induced morphological changes of isolated cochlear outer hair cells. Acta Otolaryngologica 117: 258-264.

Kaada B, Hognestad S, Havstad J (1989) Transcutaneous nerve stimulation (TNS) in tinnitus. Scandinavian Audiology 18: 211-217.

Kadner A, Viirre E, Wester DC, Walsh SF, Hestenes J, Vankov A et al. (2002) Lateral inhibition in the auditory cortex: an EEG index of tinnitus? Neuroreport 13: 443-446.

Kaldo V, Larsen HC, Andersson G (2004) Internet-based cognitive-behavioral self-help treatment of tinnitus: clinical effectiveness and predictors of outcome. American Journal of Audiology.

Kaltenbach JA, McAslin DL (1996) Increases in spontaneous activity in the dorsal cochlear nucleus following exposure to high intensity sound: a possible neural correlate of tinnitus? Auditory Neuroscience 3: 57-78.

Kaltenbach JA, Godfrey DA, McCaslin DL, Squire AB (1996) Changes in spontaneous activity and chemistry of the cochlear nucleus following intense sound exposure, In: Reich GE, Vernon JA (eds). Proceedings of the Fifth International Tinnitus Seminar 1995. Portland, Oreg: American Tinnitus Association; 429-440.

Kaltenbach JA, Heffner HE, Afman CE (1999) Effects of intense sound on spontaneous activity in the dorsal cochlear nucleus and its relation to tinnitus. In: Hazell J (ed.). Proceedings of the Sixth International Tinnitus Seminar. Cambridge: The Tinnitus and Hyperacusis Centre; 133-138.

Kandel ER, Schwartz JH, Jessel TM (eds) (2000) Principles of Neural Science. New York, NY: McGraw-Hill.

Katzenell U, Segal S (2001) Hyperacusis: review and clinical guidelines. Otology and Neurotology 22: 321-327.

Kaye JM, Marlowe FI, Ramchandani D, Berman S, Schindler B, Loscalzo G (1994) Hypnosis as an aid for tinnitus patients. Ear, Nose and Throat Journal 73: 309-315.

Kellerhals B (1999) The Swiss concept I: Tinnitus rehabilitation by training. In: Hazell J (ed.). Proceedings of the Sixth International Tinnitus Seminar. Cambridge: The Tinnitus and Hyperacusis Centre; 286-287.

Kemp DT (1978) Stimulated acoustic emissions from within the hunan auditory system. Journal of the Acoustic Society of America 64: 1386-1391.

Kemp S, George RN (1992) Diaries of tinnitus sufferers. British Journal of Audiology 26: 381-386.

Kentish RC, Crocker SR, McKenna L (2000) Children's experience of tinnitus: a preliminary survey of children presenting to a psychology department. British Journal of Audiology 34: 335-340.

Kerns RD, Turk DC, Rudy TE (1985) The West Haven–Yale multidimensional pain inventory (WHYMPI). Pain 23: 345-356.

Kessler RC, McGonagle KA, Shao S, Nelson CB, Hughes M, Eshleman S et al. (1994) Lifetime and 12-month prevalence of DSM-III-R psychiatric disorders in the United States. Archives of General Psychiatry 51: 8-19.

Kessler RC, Andrews G, Mroczek D, Ustun B, Wittchen H-U (1998) The World Health Organization composite international diagnostic interview short-form (CIDI). International Journal of Methods in Psychiatric Research 7: 171-185.

Khalfa S, Dubal S, Veuillet E, Perez-Sdiaz F, Jouvent R, Collet L (2002) Psychometric normalisation of a Hyperacusis Questionnaire. ORL 64: 436-442.

Khalil S, Ogunyemi L, Osbourne J (2002) Middle cerebral artery aneurysm presenting as isolated hyperacusis. Journal of Laryngology and Otology 116: 376-378.

Kiang NYS, Moxon EC, Levine RA (1970) Auditory-nerve activity in cats with normal and abnormal cochleas. In: Wolstenhome GE, Knight J (eds). Sensorineural Hearing Loss. London: Churchill Livingstone; 241-276.

Kihlstrom JF (1985) Hypnosis. Annual Review of Psychology 36: 385-418.

Kirsch CA, Blanchard EB, Parnes SM (1989) Psychological characteristics of individuals high and low in their ability to cope with tinnitus. Psychosomatic Medicine 51: 209-217.

Klein AJ, Armstrong BL, Greer MK, Brownn III FR (1990) Hyperacusis and otitis media in individuals with Williams syndrome. Journal of Speech and Hearing Disorders 55: 339-344.

Klockhoff I (1981) Impedance fluctuation and a 'tensor tympani syndrome'. In: Penha R, De Noronha Pizarro P (eds). Proceedings of the Fourth International Symposium on Acoustic Impedance Measurements. Lisbon: Universidade Nova de Lisaboa; 69-76.

Klockhoff I, Lindblom U (1967) Ménière's disease and hydrochlorothiazide (Dichlotride(c)) – a critical analysis of symptoms and therapeutic effects. Acta Oto-Laryngologica 63: 347-365.

Kotimaki J, Sorri M, Aantaa E, Nuutinen J (1999) Prevalence of Ménière disease in Finland. Laryngoscope 109: 748-753.

Kröner-Herwig B, Hebing G, Van Rijn-Kalkmann U, Frenzel A, Schilkowsky G, Esser G (1995) The management of chronic tinnitus. Comparison of a cognitive-behavioural group training with yoga. Journal of Psychosomatic Research 39: 153-165.

Kröner-Herwig B, Biesinger E, Goebel G, Greimel KV, Hiller W (2000) Retraining therapy for chronic tinnitus. Scandinavian Audiology 29: 67-78.

Kröner-Herwig B, Frenzel A, Fritsche G, Schilkowsky G, Esser G (2003) The management of chronic tinnitus. Comparison of an outpatient cognitive-behavioral group training to minimal-contact interventions. Journal of Psychosomatic Research 54: 381-389.

Kuk FK, Tyler RS, Russell D, Jordan H (1990) The psychometric properties of a tinnitus handicap questionnaire. Ear and Hearing 11: 434-445.

Langner G, Wallhäusser-Franke E (1999) Computer simulation of a tinnitus model based on labelling of tinnitus activity in the auditory cortex. In: Hazell J (ed.). Proceedings of the Sixth International Tinnitus seminar. Cambridge: The Tinnitus and Hyperacusis Centre; 20-25.

Langguth B, Eichhammer P, Wiegand R, Maenner P, Jacob P, Hajak G (2003) Neuronavigated rTMS in a patients with chronic tinnitus. Effects of 4 weeks of treatment. Neuroreport : 977–980.

Lazarus RS, Folkman S (1984) Coping and adaption. In: Gentry WD (ed.). Handbook of Behavioral Medicine. New York, NY: The Guilford Press; 282–325.

LeDoux JE (1998) The Emotional Brain. London: Weidenfeld & Nicholson.

Lee H, Whitman GT, Lim JG, Yi SD, Cho YW, Ying S et al. (2003) Hearing symptoms in migraneous infarction. Archives of Neurology 60: 113–116.

Lempert J (1938) Improvement in hearing in cases of otosclerosis. A new one-stage surgical technique. Archives of Otolaryngology 28: 42–97.

Leske MC (1981) Prevalence estimates of communicative disorders in the US. Language, hearing, and vestibular disorders. American Speech and Hearing Association 23: 229–237.

Lethem J, Slade PD, Troup JDG, Bentley G (1983) Outline of a fear-avoidance model of exaggerated pain perception – I. Behaviour Research and Therapy 21: 401–408.

Levin G, Fabian P, Stahle J (1988) Incidence of otosclerosis. American Journal of Otology 9: 299–301.

Levine RA (1999) Somatic modulation appears to be a fundamental attribute of tinnitus. In: Hazell J (ed.). Proceedings of the Sixth International Tinnitus Seminar. Cambridge: The Tinnitus and Hyperacusis Centre; 193–197.

Levine RA (2001) Diagnostic issues in tinnitus: a neuro-otological perspective. Seminars in Hearing 22: 23–36.

Levine RA, Kiang NYS (1995) A conversation about tinnitus. In: Vernon JA, Møller AR (eds). Mechanisms of Tinnitus. Boston, Mass: Allyn & Bacon; 149–161.

Levitin DJ, Menon V, Schmitt JE, Eliez S, White CD, Glover GH et al. (2003) Neural correlates of auditory perception in Williams syndrome: an FMRI study. Neuroimage 18: 74–82.

Lewis J, Stephens D, Huws D (1992) Suicide in tinnitus. Journal of Audiological Medicine 1: 30–37.

Lewis JE, Stephens SDG (1995) Parasuicide and tinnitus. Journal of Audiological Medicine 4: 34–39.

Lewis JE, Stephens SDG, McKenna L (1994) Tinnitus and suicide. Clinical Otolaryngology 19: 50–54.

Lewy RB (1937) Treatment of tinnitus aurium by the intravenous use of local anesthetic agents. Archives of Otolaryngology 25: 178–183.

Liedgren SR, Odkvist LM, Davis ER, Fredrickson JM (1976) Effect of marihuana on hearing. Journal of Otolaryngology 5: 233–237.

Lind O (1996) Transient evoked otoacoustic emissions and contralateral suppression in patients with unilateral tinnitus. Scandinavian Audiology 25: 167–172.

Lindberg P, Lyttkens L, Melin L, Scott B (1984) Tinnitus – incidence and handicap. Scandinavian Audiology 13: 287–291.

Linde K, Hondras M, Vickers A, ter Riet G, Melchart D (2001) Systematic reviews of complementary therapies – an annotated bibliography. Part 3: homeopathy. BMC Complementary and Alternative Medicine 1:4. (Epub)

Linton SJ, Overmeer T, Jansson M, Vlaeyen JWS, de Jong JR (2002) Graded in-vivo exposure treatment for fear-avoidant pain patients with functional disability: a case study. Cognitive Behaviour Therapy 31: 49–58.

Lockwood AH, Salvi RJ, Coad ML, Towsley ML, Wack DS, Murphy BW (1998) The functional neuroanatomy of tinnitus. Evidence for limbic system links and neural plasticity. Neurology 50: 114–120.

Lockwood AH, Wack DS, Burkard RF, Coad ML, Reyes SA, Arnold SA et al. (2001) The functional anatomy of gaze-evoked tinnitus and sustained lateral gaze. Neurology 56: 472-480.

Long GR, Tubis A (1988) Modification of spontaneous and evoked emissions and associated psychoacoustic microstructure by aspirin consumption. Journal of the Acoustical Society of America 84: 1343-1353.

Lyttkens L, Lindberg P, Scott B, Melin L (1986) Treatment of tinnitus by external electrical stimulation. Scandinavian Audiology 15: 157-164.

MacLean PD (1955) The limbic system ('visceral brain') and emotional behavior. Archives of Neurology and Psychiatry 73: 130-134.

MacLeod-Morgan C, Court J, Roberts R (1982) Cognitive restructuring: a technique for the relief of chronic tinnitus. Australian Journal of Clinical and Experimental Hypnosis 10: 27-33.

MacNaughton Jones H (1891) Subjective Noises in the Head and Ears. London: Ballière, Tindall & Cox.

Mammano F, Ashmore JF (1993) Reverse transduction measured in the isolated cochlea by laser Michelson interferometry. Nature 365: 838-841.

Marciano E, Carrabba L, Giannini P, Sementina C, Verde P, Bruno C et al. (2003) Psychiatric comorbidity in a population of outpatients affected by tinnitus. International Journal of Audiology 42: 4-9.

Marks NJ, Emery P, Onisphorou C (1984) A controlled trial of acupuncture in tinnitus. Journal of Laryngology and Otology 98: 1103-1109.

Marks NJ, Karl H, Onisiphorou C (1985) A controlled trial of hypnotherapy in tinnitus. Clinical Otolaryngology 10: 43-46.

Marlowe FI (1973) Effective treatment of tinnitus through hypnotherpy. American Journal of Clinical Hypnosis 15: 162-165.

Marriage J, Barnes NM (1995) Is central hyperacusis a symptom of 5-hydroxytryptamine (5-HT) dysfunction? Journal of Laryngology and Otology 109: 915-921.

Martin K, Snashall S (1994) Children presenting with tinnitus: a retrospective study. British Journal of Audiology 28: 111-115.

Martin W (1995) Spectral analysis of brain activity in the study of tinnitus. In: Vernon JA, Møller AR (eds). Mechanisms of Tinnitus. London: Allyn & Bacon; 163-180.

Mason J, Rogerson D (1995) Client-centered hypnotherapy for tinnitus: who is likely to benefit? American Journal of Clinical Hypnosis 37: 294-299.

Mason JDT, Rogerson DR, Butler JD (1996) Client centered hypnotherapy in the management of tinnitus – is it better than counselling? Journal of Laryngology and Otology 110: 117-120.

Matsuhira T, Yamashita K, Yasuda M (1992) Estimation of the loudness of tinnitus from matching tests. British Journal of Audiology 26: 387-395.

Maurizi M, Ottaviani F, Paludetti G, Almadori G, Tassoni A (1985) Contribution to the differentiation of peripheral versus central tinnitus via auditory brain stem response evaluation. Audiology 24: 207-216.

McCombe A, Baguley D, Coles R, McKenna L, McKinney C, Windle-Taylor P (2001) Guidelines for the grading of tinnitus severity: the results of a working group commissioned by the British Association of Otolaryngologists, Head and Neck Surgeons. Clinical Otolaryngology 26: 388-393.

McFadden D (1982) Tinnitus. Facts, Theories, and Treatments. Washington, DC: National Academy Press.

McFadden D, Pasanen EG (1994) Otoacoustic emissions and quinine sulfate. Journal of the Acoustical Society of America 95: 3460-3474.

McKee GJ, Stephens SDG (1992) An investigation of normally hearing subjects with tinnitus. Audiology 31: 313–317.

McKenna L (1987) Goal planning in audiological rehabilitation. British Journal of Audiology 21: 5–11.

McKenna L (1997) Audiological disorders: psychological state and cognitive functioning. Unpublished doctoral thesis. London: The City University.

McKenna L (2000) Tinnitus and insomnia. In: Tyler RS (ed.). Tinnitus Handbook. San Diego, Calif: Singular, Thomson Learning; 59–84.

McKenna L (2004) Models of tinnitus suffering and treatment: compared and contrasted. Audiological Medicine 2: 41–53.

McKenna L, Hallam R (1999) A neuropsychological study of concentration problems in tinnitus patients. In: Hazell J (ed.). Proceedings of the Sixth International Tinnitus Seminar. Cambridge: The Tinnitus and Hyperacusis Centre; 108–113.

McKenna L, Daniel HC (2003) The psychological management of tinnitus related insomnia. In: Tyler R (ed.). Tinnitus Management.

McKenna L, Hallam RS, Hinchcliffe R (1991) The prevalence of psychological disturbance in neuro-otology outpatients. Clinical Otolaryngology 16: 452–456.

McKenna L, Hallam RS, Shurlock L (1996) Cognitive functioning in tinnitus patients. In: Reich GE, Vernon JA (eds). Proceedings of the Fifth International Tinnitus Seminar 1995. Portland, Oreg: American Tinnitus Association; 589–595.

McKinney CJ, Hazell JWP, Graham RL (1999) The effects of hearing loss on tinnitus. In: Hazell J (ed.). Proceedings of the Sixth International Tinnitus Seminar. Cambridge: The Tinnitus and Hyperacusis Centre; 407–414.

McNeill C (ed.) (1993) Temporomandibular Disorders. Guidelines for Classification, Assessment, and Management. Chicago, Ill: Quintessence.

Meikle MB, Greist SE (1989) Gender-based differences in characteristics of tinnitus. Hearing Journal 42: 68–76.

Meikle MB, Greist SE (1992) Asymmetry in tinnitus perceptions. Factors that may account for the higher prevalence of left-sided tinnitus. In: Aran J-M, Dauman R (eds). Tinnitus '91. Proceedings of the Fourth International Tinnitus Seminar. Amsterdam: Kugler Publications; 231–237.

Meikle MB, Taylor-Walsh E (1984) Characteristics of tinnitus and related observations in over 1800 tinnitus clinic patients. Journal of Laryngology and Otology (Suppl.) 9: 17–21.

Melcher JR, Sigalosky IS, Guinan JJ, Levine RA (2000) Lateralized tinnitus studied with functional magnetic resonance imaging: abnormal inferior colliculus activation. Journal of Neurophysiology 83: 1058–1072.

Melin L, Scott B, Lindberg P, Lyttkens L (1987) Hearing aids and tinnitus – an experimental group study. British Journal of Audiology 21: 91–97.

Meric C, Gartner M, Collet L, Chéry-Croze S (1998) Psychopathological profile of tinnitus sufferers: evidence concerning the relationship between tinnitus features and impact on life. Audiology and Neuro-Otology 3: 240–252.

Mihail RC, Crowley JM, Walden BE, Fishburne J, Reinwall JE, Zajtchuck JT (1988) The tricyclic trimipramine in the treatment of tinnitus. Annals of Otology, Rhinology and Laryngology 97: 120–123.

Miller JJ (1985) CRC Handbook of Ototoxicity. Roca Baton, Fla: CRC Press.

Mills RP, Cherry JR (1984) Subjective tinnitus in children with otological disorders. International Journal of Pediatric Otorhinolaryngology 7: 21–27.

Mills RP, Albert DM, Brain C.E (1986) Tinnitus in childhood. Clinical Otolaryngology 11: 431–434.

Mimeault V, Morin CM (1999) Self-help treatment for insomnia: bibliotherapy with and without professional guidance. Journal of Consulting and Clinical Psychology 67: 511-519.

Min SK, Lee BO (1997) Laterality in somatization. Psychosomatic Medicine 59: 236-240.

Minton JP (1923) Tinnitus and its relation to nerve deafness with application of the masking effect of pure tones. Physical Review 22: 506-509.

Mirz F, Pedersen CB, Ishizu K, Johannsen P, Ovesen T, Sõdkilde-Jõrgensen H et al. (1999a) Positron emission tomography of cortical centres of tinnitus. Hearing Research 134: 133-144.

Mirz F, Stødkilde-Jørgensen H, Pedersen CB (1999b) Evidence of cortical networks subserving the perception of tinnitus: an fMRI study. Neuroimage 9: S794.

Mirz F, Gjedde A, Sõdkilde-Jõrgensen H, Pedersen CB (2000) Functional brain imaging of tinnitus-like perception induced by aversive auditory stimuli. Neuroreport 11: 633-637.

Mirz F, Mortensen M, Gjedde A, Pedersen CB (2002) Positron emission tomography of tinnitus suppression by cochlear implantation. In: Patuzzi R (ed.). Proceedings of the Seventh International Tinnitus Seminar. Freemantle: University of Western Australia; 136-140.

Mirz F, Zachariae R, Andersen SE, Nielsen AG, Johansen LV, Bjerring P et al. (1999c) The low-power laser in the treatment of tinnitus. Clinical Otolaryngology 24: 346-354.

Mitchell CR, Vernon JA, Creedon TA (1993) Measuring tinnitus parameters: loudness, pitch, and maskability. Journal of the American Academy of Audiology 4: 139-151.

Mitchell PL, Moffat DA, Fallside F (1984) Computer-aided tinnitus characterization. Clinical Otolaryngology 9: 35-42.

Moffat DA, Hardy DG, Irving RM, Viani L, Bey GJ, Baguley DM (1995) Referral patterns in vestibular Schwannomas. Clinical Otolaryngology 20: 80-83.

Møller AR (1984) Pathophysiology of tinnitus. Annals of Otology 93: 39-44.

Møller AR (1997) Similarities between chronic pain and tinnitus. American Journal of Otology 18: 577-585.

Møller AR (1998) Vascular compression of cranial nerves. 1: History of the microvascular decompression operation. Neurological Research 20: 727-731.

Møller AR, Møller MB, Yokota M (1992) Some forms of tinnitus may involve the extralemniscal auditory pathway. Laryngoscope 102: 1165-1171.

Møller MB, Møller AR, Jannetta PJ, Ito HD (1993). Vascular decompression surgery for severe tinnitus: selection criteria and results. Laryngoscope 103: 421-427.

Moore BC.J (1998) Cochlear Hearing Loss. London: Whurr Publishers.

Morin CM (1993) Insomnia. Psychological Assessment and Management. New York, NY: Guilford Press.

Morin CM, Culbert JP, Schwartz SM (1994) Nonpharmacological interventions for insomnia: a meta-analysis of treatment efficacy. American Journal of Psychiatry 151: 1172-1180.

Morin CM, Hauri PJ, Espie CA, Spielman AJ, Buysse DJ, Bootzon RR (1999) Nonpharmacological treatment of chronic insomnia. Sleep 22: 1134-1156.

Morrison AW, Bundey SE (1970) The inheritance of otosclerosis. Journal of Laryngology and Otology 84: 921-932.

Morrison GA, Sterkers JM (1996) Unusual presentations of acoustic tumours. Clinical Otolaryngology 21: 80-83.

Mühlnickel W, Elbert T, Taub E, Flor H (1998) Reorganization of the auditory cortex in tinnitus. Proceedings of the National Academy of Science 95: 10 340-10 343.

Murai K, Tyler RS, Harker LA, Stouffer JL (1992) Review of pharmacological treatment of tinnitus. American Journal of Otology 13: 454-464.

Murtagh DRR, Greenwood KM (1995) Identifying effective psychological treatments for insomnia. Journal of Consulting and Clinical Psychology 63: 79-89.

Nagel D, Drexel MKA (1989) Epidemiologische untersuchungen zum tinnitus aurium. Auris Nasus Larynx 16: S23-S31.

Nakashima T, Ueda H, Misawa H, Suzuki T, Tominaga M, Ito A et al. (2002) Transmeatal low-power laser irridation for tinnitus. Otology and Neurootology 23: 296-300.

Nebeska M, Rubinstein B, Wenneberg B (1999) Influence of acupuncture on tinnitus in patients with signs and symptoms of temporomandibular disorders: a placebo-controlled study. In: Hazell J (ed.). Proceedings of the Sixth International Tinnitus Seminar. Cambridge: The Tinnitus and Hyperacusis Centre; 575-577.

Nelken I, Young ED (1996) Why do cats need a dorsal cochlear nucleus? Journal of Basic Clinical Physiology and Pharmacology 7: 199-220.

Nelting M, Rienhoff NK, Hesse G, Lamparter U (2002) The assessment of subjective distress related to hyperacusis with a self-rating quaetionnaire on hypersensitivity to sound. Laryngorhinootlogie 81: 32-34.

Newman CW, Weinstein BE, Jacobson GP, Hug GA (1990) The hearing handicap inventory for adults: psychometric adequacy and audiometric correlates. Ear and Hearing 11: 430-433.

Newman CW, Jacobson GP, Spitzer JB (1996) Development of the tinnitus handicap inventory. Archives of Otolaryngology, Head, and Neck Surgery 122: 143-148.

Newman CW, Jacobson GP, Hug GA, Sandridge SA (1997) Perceived hearing handicap of patients with unilateral or mild hearing loss. Annals of Otology, Rhinology & Laryngology 106: 210-214.

Newman CW, Sandridge SA, Jacobson G (1998) Psychometric adequacy of the Tinnitus Handicap Inventory (THI) for evaluating treatment outcome. Journal of the American Academy of Audiology 9: 153-160.

Nields JA, Fallon BA, Jastreboff P (1999) Carbamazepine in the treatment of Lyme disease-induced hyperacusis. Journal of Neuropsychiatry and Clinical Neuroscience 11: 97-99.

Nieschalk M, Hustert B, Stoll W (1998) Auditory reaction times in patients with chronic tinnitus with normal hearing. American Journal of Otology 19: 611-618.

Noble W (1998) Self-assessment of Hearing and Related Functions. London: Whurr Publishers.

Noble W (2000) Self-reports about tinnitus and about cochlear implants. Ear and Hearing 21: 50S-59S.

Nodar RH (1972) Tinnitus aurium in school age children. Journal of Auditory Research 12: 133-135.

Nodar RH (1996) Tinnitus reclassified: new oil in an old lamp. Otolaryngology, Head, and Neck Surgery 114: 582-585.

Nondahl DM, Cruickshanks KJ, Wiley TL, Klein R, Klein BEK, Tweed TS (2002) Prevalence and 5-year incidence of tinnitus among older adults: the epidemiology of hearing loss study. Journal of the American Academy of Audiology 13: 323-331.

Norcross JC, Santrock JW, Campbell LF, Smith TP, Sommer R, Zuckerman EL (2000) Authoritative Guide to Self-help Resources in Mental Health. New York, NY: Guilford Press.

Norena A, Cransac H, Chéry-Croze S (1999) Towards an objectification by classification of tinnitus. Clinical Neurophysiology 110: 666-675.

Ochi K, Ohasi T, Kinoshita H (1997) Serum zinc levels in patients with tinnitus and the effect of zinc treatment. Annals of Otology, Rhinology and Laryngology (Japan) 100: 915-919.

Ochi K, Kinoshita H, Kenmochi M, Nishino H, Ohasi T (2003) Zinc defiency and tinnitus. Auris Nasus Larynx 30: 25-28.

Ogata Y, Sekitani T, Moriya K, Watanabe K (1993) Biofeedback therapy in the treatment of tinnitus. Auris Nasus Larynx 20: 95-101.

Ogles BM, Lunnen KM, Bonesteel K (2001) Clinical significance: history, application, and current practice. Clinical Psychology Review 21: 421-446.

Oort H (1918) Uber die verastellung des nervus octavus bei sautetieren. Anat Anz 51: 272-280.

Öst L-G (1987) Applied relaxation: description of a coping technique and review of controlled studies. Behaviour Research and Therapy 25: 379-409.

Öst L-G (1997) Rapid treatments of specific phobias. In: Davey GCL (ed.) Phobias. A handbook of theory research and treatment. Chichester: John Wiley & Sons; 227-246.

Paaske PB, Pedersen CB, Kjems G, Sam I (1991) Zinc in the management of tinnitus. Placebo-controlled trial. Annals of Otology Rhinology and Laryngology 100: 647-649.

Palmer KT, Griffin MJ, Syddall HE, Davis A, Pannett B, Coggon D (2002) Occupational exposure to noise and the attributable burden of hearing difficulties in Great Britain. Occupational and Environmental Medicine 59: 634-639.

Pantev C, Hoke M, Lütkenhöner B, Lehnertz K, Kumpf W (1989) Tinnitus remission objectified by neuromagnetic measurements. Hearing Research 40: 216-264.

Papez JW (1937) A proposed mechanism of emotion. Archives of Neurology and Psychiatry 38: 725-743.

Park J, White AR, Ernst E (2000) Efficacy of acupuncture as a treatment for tinnitus. A systematic review. Archives of Otolaryngology – Head and Neck Surgery 126: 489-492.

Parving A, Hein HO, Suadicani B, Ostri B, Gyntelberg F (1993) Epidemiology of hearing disorders. Scandinavian Audiology 22: 101-107.

Pavlov IP (1927) Conditioned Reflexes. New York, NY: Oxford University Press.

Pearson MM, Barnes LJ (1950) Objective tinnitus aurium: report of two cases with good results after hypnosis. Journal of Philadelphia General Hospital 1: 134-138.

Penner MJ (1983) Variability in matches to subjective tinnitus. Journal of Speech and Hearing Research 26: 263-267.

Penner MJ (1986) Magnitude estimation and the 'paradoxical' loudness of tinnitus. Journal of Speech and Hearing Research 29: 407-412.

Penner MJ (1987) Masking of tinnitus and central masking. Journal of Speech and Hearing Research 30: 147-152.

Penner MJ (1993) Synthesizing tinnitus from sine waves. Journal of Speech and Hearing Research 36: 1300-1305.

Penner MJ (1996) Rating the annoyance of synthesized tinnitus. International Tinnitus Journal 2: 3-7.

Penner MJ, Burns EM (1987) The dissociation of SOAEs and tinnitus. Journal of Speech and Hearing Research 30: 396-403.

Penner MJ, Bilger RC (1988) Adaption and the masking of tinnitus. Journal of Speech and Hearing Research 32: 339-346.

Penner MJ, Coles RRA (1992) Aspirin as a palliative for SOAE-caused tinnitus. British Journal of Audiology 26: 91-96.

Penner MJ, Jastreboff PJ (1996) Tinnitus: psychophysical observations in humans and an animal model. In: Van De Water TR, Popper AN, Fay RR (eds). Clinical Aspects of Hearing. New York, NY: Springer Verlag; 258-304.

Penner MJ, Klafter EJ (1992) Measures of tinnitus: step size, matches to imagined tones, and masking patterns. Tinnitus Mätning Vägning 13: 410-416.

Penner MJ, Brauth S, Hood L (1981) The temporal course of the masking of tinnitus as a basis for inferring its origin. Journal of Speech and Hearing Research 24: 257-261.

Perlman HB (1938) Hyperacusis. Annals of Otology, Rhinology and Laryngology 47: 947–953.

Persons JB, Davidson J (2001) Cognitive-behavioral case formulation. In: Dobson KS (ed.). Handbook of Cognitive-behavioral Therapies. New York, NY: Guilford Press; 86–110.

Persons JB, Davidson J, Tompkins MA (2001) Essential Components of Cognitive-behavior Therapy for Depression. Washington, DC: American Psychological Association.

Peters ML, Vlaeyen JWS, van Drunen C (2000) Do fibromyalgia patients display hypervigilance for innocuous somatosensory stimuli? Application of a body scanning reaction time paradigm. Pain 86: 283–292.

Phillips DP, Carr MM (1998) Disturbances of loudness perception. Journal of the American Academy of Audiology 9: 371–379.

Philips HC, Rachman S (1996) The Psychological Management of Pain. New York, NY: Springer.

Pilgramm M, Rychlick R, Lebisch H, Siedentop H, Goebel G, Kirchoff D (1999) In: Hazell J (ed.). Proceedings of the Sixth International Tinnitus Seminar. Cambridge: The Tinnitus and Hyperacusis Centre; 64–67.

Pinchoff RJ, Burkard RF, Salvi RJ, Coad ML, Lockwood AH (1998) Modulation of tinnitus by voluntary jaw movements. American Journal of Otology 19: 785–789.

Plath P, Olivier J (1995) Results of combined low-power laser therapy and extracts of Ginkgo Biloba in cases of sensorineural hearing loss and tinnitus. Advances in Otorhinolaryngology 49: 101–104.

Podoshin L, Ben-David Y, Fradis M, Gerstel R, Felner H (1991) Idiopathic subjective tinnitus treated by biofeedback, acupuncture and drug therapy. Ear, Nose and Throat Journal 70: 284–289.

Pratt H (2003) Human auditory electrophysiology. In: Luxon L, Furman JM, Martini M, Stephens D (eds). Textbook of Audiological Medicine. Clinical Aspects of Hearing and Balance. London: Martin Dunitz; 271–287.

Prezant TR, Agapian JV, Bohlman MC, Bu X, Oztas S, Qiu WQ (1993) Mitochondrial ribosomal RNA mutation associated with both antibiotic-induced and non–syndromic deafness. Nature Genetics 4: 289–294.

Puel JL, Bobbin RP, Fallon M (1990) Salicylate, mefenamate, meclofenamate and quinine on cochlear potential. Otolaryngology, Head and Neck Surgery 102: 66–73.

Puel JL (1995) Chemical synaptic transmission in the cochlea. Progress in Neurobiology 47: 449–476.

Pugh R, Budd RJ, Stephens SDG (1995) Patients' reports of the effect of alcohol on tinnitus. British Journal of Audiology 29: 279–283.

Pugh R, Stephens SDG, Budd R (2004). The contribution of spouse responses and marital satisfaction to the experience of chronic tinnitus. Audiological Medicine 2: 60–73.

Pulec JL (1967) Abnormally patent eustachian tubes: treatment with injection of poly-tetrafluoroethylene (teflon) paste. Laryngoscope 77: 1543–1554.

Pulec JL (1995) Cochlear nerve section for intractable tinnitus. Ear Nose and Throat Journal 74: 468–476.

Quaranta A, Assennato G, Sallustio V (1996) Epidemiology of hearing problems among adults in Italy. Scandinavian Audiology 25 (Suppl. 42): 7–11.

Quaranta N, Wagstaff S, Baguley DM (2004) Tinnitus and cochlear implantation. International Journal of Audiology 43(5): 245–251.

Quick CA (1973) Chemical and drug effects on the inner ear. In: Paparella MM, Shumrick DA (eds). Otolaryngology, Vol. 2. Philadelphia, Pa: WB Saunders; 392.

Rasmussen GL (1946) The olivary peduncle and other fiber projections of the superior olivary complex. Journal of Comparative Neurology 99: 61–74.

Rauschecker JP (1999) Auditory cortical plasticity: a comparison with other sensory systems. Trends in Neuroscience 22: 74-80.

Rechtshaffen A, Siegel J (2000) Sleep and dreaming. In: Kandel ER, Schwartz JH, Jessel TM (eds). Principles of Neural Science. New York, NY: McGraw-Hill; 936-947.

Reed GF (1960) An audiometric study of two hundered cases of subjective tinnitus. Archives of Otolaryngology 71: 94-104.

Reed HT, Meltzer J, Crews P, Norris CH, Quine DB, Guth PS (1985). Amino-oxyacetic acid as a palliative in tinnitus. Archives of Otolaryngology, Head and Neck Surgery 111: 803-805.

Reich G, Johnson R (1984) Personality characteristics of tinnitus patients. Journal of Laryngology and Otology 97: 228-232.

Reiss S, Peterson RA, Gurksy DM, McNally RJ (1986) Anxiety sensitivity, anxiety frequency and the prediction of fearfulness. Behaviour Research and Therapy 34: 1-8.

Reyes S, Salvi R, Burkard R, Coad M, Wack D, Galantowicz P et al. (2002) Brain imaging of the effects of lidocaine on tinnitus. Hearing Research 171: 43-50.

Ringdahl A, Eriksson-Mangold M, Andersson G (1998) Psychometric evaluation of the Gothenburg Profile for measurement of experienced hearing disability and handicap: applications with new hearing aid candidates and experienced hearing aid users. British Journal of Audiology 32: 375-385.

Risey J, Briner W, Guth PS, Norris CH (1989) The superiority of the Goodwin procedure over the traditional procedure in measuring the loudness level of tinnitus. Ear and Hearing 10: 318-322.

Robertson D, Irvine DRF (1989) Plasticity of frequency organization in auditory cortex of guinea pigs with partial unilateral deafness. Journal of Comparative Neurology 282: 456-471.

Robinson PJ, Hazell JWP (1989) Patulous Eustachian tube syndrome: the relationship with sensorineural deafness: treatment by Eustachian tube diathermy. Journal of Laryngology and Otology 103: 739-742.

Ronis M (1984) Alcohol and dietary influence on tinnitus. Journal of Laryngology and Otology 98 (Suppl. 9): 242-246.

Rosen S (1953) Mobilization of the stapes to restore hearing in otosclerosis. New York Journal of Medicine 53: 2650-2653.

Rosenberg S, Silverstein H, Rowan PT, Olds MJ (1998) Effect of melatonin on tinnitus. Laryngoscope 108: 305-310.

Rosenhall U, Axelsson A (1995) Auditory brainstem response latencies in patients with tinnitus. Scandinavian Audiology 24: 97-100.

Rosenhall U, Karlsson A-K (1991) Tinnitus in old age. Scandinavian Audiology 20: 165-171.

Rosenstiel AK, Keefe FJ (1983) The use of coping strategies in chronic low back pain patients: relationship to patient characteristics and current adjustment. Pain 17: 33-44.

Roth A, Fonagy P (1996) What Works for Whom? A Critical Review of Psychotherapy Research. New York, NY: Guilford Press.

Rubinstein B (1993) Tinnitus and craniomandibular disorders – is there a link? Swedish Dental Journal 95 (Suppl.): 95; 1-46.

Rubinstein B, Carlsson GE (1987) Effects of stomatognathic treatment on tinnitus: a retrospective study. Journal of Craniomandibular Practice 5: 254-259.

Rubinstein B, Axelsson A, Carlsson GE (1990) Prevalence of signs and symptoms of craniomandibular disorders in tinnitus patients. Journal of Craniomandibular Disorders and Facial Oral Pain 4: 186-192.

Rubinstein B, Österberg T, Rosenhall U (1992) Longitudinal fluctuations in tinnitus as reported by an elderly population. Journal of Audiological Medicine 1: 149-155.

Rubinstein B, Ahlqwist M, Bengtsson C (1996) Hyperacusis, headache, temporo-mandibular disorders and amalgam fillings – an epidemiological study. In: Reich GE, Vernon JA (eds). Proceedings of the Fifth International Tinnitus Seminar 1995. Portland, Oreg: American Tinnitus Association; 657–658.

Rubinstein JT, Tyler RS, Johnson A, Brown CJ (2003) Electrical suppression of tinnitus with high-rate pulse trains. Otology and Neurotology 24: 478–485.

Russo JE, Katon WJ, Sullivan MD, Clark MR, Buchwald D (1994) Severity of somatization and its relationship to psychiatric disorders and personality. Psychosomatics 35: 546–556.

Sackett DL, Strauss SE, Richardson WS, Rosenberg W, Haynes RB (2000) Evidence-based medicine. How to practice and teach EBM. Edinburgh: Churchill Livingstone.

Sadlier M, Stephens SDG (1995) An approach to the audit of tinnitus management. Journal of Laryngology and Otology 109: 826–829.

Saeed SR, Brookes GB (1993) The use of clostridium botulinum toxin in palatal myoclonus. A preliminary report. Journal of Laryngology and Otology 107: 208–210.

Sahley TL, Nodar RH (2001) A biochemical model of peripheral tinnitus. Hearing Research 152: 43–54.

Sahley TL, Nodar RH, Musiek FE (1997) Efferent Auditory System: Structure and Function. San Diego, Calif: Singular.

Saltzman M, Ersner MS (1947) A hearing aid for the relief of tinnitus aurium. Laryngoscope 57: 358–366.

Salvi RJ, Wang J, Powers NL (1996) Plasticity and reorganization in the auditory brainstem: implications for tinnitus. In: Reich GE, Vernon JE (eds). Proceedings of the Fifth International Tinnitus Seminar 1995. Portland, Oreg: American Tinnitus Association; 457–466.

Salvi RJ, Lockwood AH, Burkard R (2000) Neural plasticity and tinnitus. In: Tyler RS (ed.). Tinnitus Handbook. San Diego, Calif: Singular, Thomson Learning; 123–148.

Sammeth CA, Preves DA, Brandy WT (2000) Hyperacusis: case studies and evaluation of electronic loudness suppression devices as a treatment approach. Scandinavian Audiology 29: 28–36.

Sanchez L, Stephens D (1997) A tinnitus problem questionnaire. Ear and Hearing 18: 210–217.

Sanchez TG, Balbani APS, Bittar RSM, Bento RF, Camara J (1999) Lidocaine test: effect in patients with tinnitus and relation to the treatment with carbamazepine. In: Hazell JWPH (ed.). Proceedings of the Sixth International Tinnitus Seminar. Cambridge: The Tinnitus and Hyperacusis Centre; 538–542.

Saper CB (2000) Brain stem, reflexive behavior, and the cranial nerves. In: Kandel ER, Schwartz JH, Jessel TM (eds). Principles of Neural Science. New York, NY: McGraw-Hill; 873–909.

Sataloff RT, Mandel S, Muscal E, Park CH, Rosen DC, Kim SM et al. (1996) Single-photon-emission computed tomography (SPECT) in neurotologic assessment: a preliminary report. American Journal of Otology 17: 909–916.

Scharf BJM, Chays A (1997) On the role of the olivocochlear bundle in hearing: 16 case studies. Hearing Research 103: 101–122.

Scheier MF, Carver CS (1985) Optimism, coping, and health: assessment and implications of generalized outcome expectancies. Health Psychology 4: 219–247.

Schilter B, Jäger B, Heermann R, Lamprecht F (2000) Medikamentöse und psychologische therapien bei chronischem subjektivem tinnitus. (Meta-analysis on the effectiveness of pharmacological and psychological treatments for chronic tinnitus aurium.) HNO 48: 589–597.

Schloth E, Zwicker E (1983) Mechanical and acoustical influences on spontaneous oto-acoustic emissions. Hearing Research 11: 285-293.

Schmidtt C, Patak M, Kröner-Herwig B (2000) Stress and the onset of sudden hearing loss and tinnitus. International Tinnitus Journal 6: 41-49.

Schmidtt C, Kröner-Herwig B (2002) Comparison of tinnitus coping training and TRT: are they superior to education? In: Patuzzi R (ed.). Proceedings of the Seventh International Tinnitus Seminar. Freemantle: University of Western Australia; 272-276.

Schneer HI (1956) Psychodynamics of tinnitus. Psychoanalytic Quarterly 25: 72-78.

Schuknecht HF (1993) Pathology of the Ear (second edition). Philadelphia, Pa: Lea & Febiger.

Schulman A (1985) External electrical stimulation in tinnitus control. American Journal of Otology 6: 110-115.

Schulman A (1995) A final common pathway for tinnitus – the medial temporal lobe system. International Tinnitus Journal 1: 115-126.

Schulman A (1997) Epidemiology of tinnitus. In: Shulman A, Aran J-M, Feldmann H, Tonndorf J, Vernon JA (eds). Tinnitus. Diagnosis and Treatment. San Diego, Calif: Singular Publishing.

Schwaber MK, Whetsell WO (1992) Cochleovestibular nerve compression syndrome. II. Histopathology and theory of pathophysiology. Laryngoscope 102: 1030-1036.

Schwartz B (1989) Psychology of Learning and Behavior. New York, NY: WW Norton & Co.

Schwartz N (1999) Self-reports. How the questions shape the answers. American Psychologist 54: 93-105.

Scogin F, Bynum J, Stephens G, Calhoon S (1990) Efficacy of self-administered treatment programs: meta-analytic review. Professional Psychology: Research and Practice 21: 42-47.

Scott B (1993) A Graded Exposure Treatment for Patients with Hyperacusis. Paper presented at the 19th Annual Convention of the Association for Behavior Analysis, Chicago, Ill, May.

Scott B, Lindberg P (2000) Psychological profile and somatic complaints between help-seeking and non-help-seeking tinnitus subjects. Psychosomatics 41: 347-352.

Scott B, Lindberg P, Melin L, Lyttkens L (1985) Psychological treatment of tinnitus. An experimental group study. Scandinavian Audiology 14: 223-230.

Scott B, Lindberg P, Melin L, Lyttkens L (1990) Predictors of tinnitus discomfort, adaption and subjective loudness. British Journal of Audiology 24: 51-62.

Seely DR, Quigley SM, Langman AW (1996) Ear candles – efficacy and safety. Laryngoscope 10: 1226-1229.

Seidman MD, Babu S (2003) Alternative medications and other treatments for tinnitus: facts from fiction. Otolaryngologic Clinics of North America 36: 359-382.

Seligman MEP (1995) The effectiveness of psychotherapy. The consumer reports study. American Psychologist 50: 965-974.

Seltzer Z, Devor M (1979) Ephaptic transmission in chronically damaged peripheral nerves. Neurology 29: 1061-1064.

Senge PM (1990) The Fifth Discipline. London: Random House.

Shailer MJ, Tyler RS, Coles RRA (1981) Critical masking bands for sensorineural tinnitus. Scandinavian Audiology 10: 157-162.

Shambaugh GE (1986) Zinc for tinnitus, imbalance and hearing loss in the elderly. American Journal of Otology 7: 476-477.

Shea JJ (1958) Fenestration of the oval window. Annals of Otology, Rhinology and Laryngology 67: 932-951.

Sheldrake JB, Hazell JWP, Graham RL (1999) Results of tinnitus retraining therapy. In: Hazell J (ed.). Proceedings of the Sixth International Tinnitus Seminar. Cambridge: The Tinnitus and Hyperacusis Centre; 292–296.

Shergill SS, Brammer MJ, Williams SCR, Murray RM, McGuire PK (2000) Mapping auditory hallucinations in schizophrenia using functional magnetic resonance imaging. Archives of General Psychiatry 57: 1033–1038.

Shiomi Y, Takahashi H, Honjo I, Kojima H, Naito Y, Fujiki N (1997) Efficacy of transmeatal low power laser irradiation on tinnitus: a preliminary report. Auris Nasus Larynx 24: 39–42.

Silberstein SD (1995) Migraine symptoms: results of a survey of self-reported migraineurs. Headache 35: 387–396.

Silberstein SD, Saper JR, Freitag FG (2001) Migrane: diagnosis and treatment. In: Silberstein SD, Lipton RB, Dalessio DJ (eds). Woolffs Headache and Other Head Pain (seventh edition). Oxford: Oxford University Press; 121–237.

Simpson JJ, Davies WE (1999) Recent advanced in the pharmacological treatment of tinnitus. Trends in Pharmacological Science 20: 12–18.

Simpson JJ, Davies WE (2000) A review of evidence in support of a role for 5-HT in the perception of tinnitus. Hearing Research 145: 1–7.

Simpson JJ, Gilbert AM, Weiner GM, Davies WE (1999). The assessment of lamotrigine, an antiepileptic drug in the treatment of tinnitus. American Journal of Otology 20: 627–631.

Simpson JJ, Donaldson I, Davies WE (1998) Use of homeopathy in the treatment of tinnitus. British Journal of Audiology 32: 227–233.

Simpson RB, Nedzelski JM, Barber HO, Thomas MR (1988) Psychiatric diagnoses in patients with psychogenic dizziness or severe tinnitus. Journal of Otolaryngology 17: 325–330.

Sismanis A (1987) Otologic manifestations of benign intracranial hypertension syndrome: diagnosis and management. Laryngoscope 97 (Suppl. 42): 1–17.

Sismanis A, Smoker WRK (1994) Pulsatile tinnitus: recent advances in diagnosis. Laryngoscope 104: 681–687.

Smith P, Coles R (1987) Epidemiology of tinnitus: an update. In: Feldman H (ed.). Proceedings of the Third International Tinnitus Seminar. Karlsruhe: Harsch Verlag; 147–153.

Smith PA, Parrr VM, Lutman ME, Coles RRA (1991) Comparative study of four noise spectra as potential tinnitus maskers. British Journal of Audiology 25: 25–34.

Sood SK, Coles RRA (1988) Hyperacusis and phonophobia in tinnitus patients. British Journal of Audiology 22: 228.

Spitzer JB, Ventry IM (1980) Central auditory dysfunction among chronic alcoholics. Archives of Otolaryngology 106: 224–229.

Stacey JSG (1980) Apparent total control of severe bilateral tinnitus by masking, using hearing aids. British Journal of Audiology 14: 59–60.

Staffen W, Biesinger E, Trinka E, Ladurner G (1999) The effect of lidocaine on chronic tinnitus: a quantative cerebral perfusion study. Audiology 38: 53–57.

Stahle J, Stahle C, Arenberg IK (1978) Incidence of Ménière's disease. Archives of Otolaryngology 104: 99–102.

Stansfeld SA (1992) Noise, noise sensitivity and psychiatric disorder: epidemiological and psychophysiological studies. Psychological Medicine Monograph Supplement 22: 1–44.

Stansfeld SA, Clark CA, Jenkins LM, Tarnopolsky A (1985) Sensitivity to noise in a community sample. 1. The measurement of psychiatric disorder and personality. Psychological Medicine 15: 243–254.

Staples SL (1996) Human response to environmental noise. American Psychologist 51: 143-150.

Steigerwald DP, Verne SV, Young D (1996) A retrospective evaluation of the impact of temporomandibular joint arthroscopy on the symptoms of headache, neck pain, shoulder pain, dizziness, and tinnitus. Journal of Craniomandibular Practise 14: 46-54.

Stephens D (1999) Detrimental effects of alcohol on tinnitus. Clinical Otolaryngology 24: 114-116.

Stephens SDG (1987) Historical aspects of tinnitus. In: Hazell JWPH (ed.). Tinnitus. London: Churchill Livingstone; 1-19.

Stephens D (2000) A history of tinnitus. In: Tyler RS (ed.). Tinnitus Handbook. San Diego, Calif: Singular, Thomson Learning; 437-448.

Stephens SDG, Corcoran AL (1985) A controlled study of tinnitus masking. British Journal of Audiology 19: 159-167.

Stephens SDG, Blegvad B, Krogh HJ (1977) The value of some suprathreshold auditory measures. Scandinavian Audiology 6: 213-221.

Stephens SDG, Hallam RS (1985) The Crown-Crisp Experiental Index in patients complaining of tinnitus. British Journal of Audiology 19: 151-158.

Stephens SDG, Hallam RS, Jakes SC (1986) Tinnitus: a management model. Clinical Otolaryngology 11: 227-238.

Stouffer JL, Tyler RS (1990) Characterization of tinnitus by tinnitus patients. Journal of Speech and Hearing Research 55: 493-453.

Stouffer JL, Tyler RS (1992) Ratings of psychological changes pre- and post-tinnitus onset. In: Aran J-M, Dauman R (eds). Tinnitus '91. Proceedings of the Fourth International Tinnitus Seminar. Amsterdam: Kugler Publications; 449-452.

Stouffer JL, Tyler RS, Kileny PR, Dalzell LE (1991) Tinnitus as a function of duration and etiology: counselling implications. American Journal of Otolaryngology 12: 188-194.

Stouffer JL, Tyler RS, Booth JC, Buckrell B (1992) Tinnitus in normal-hearing and hearing-impaired children. In: Aran J-M, Dauman R (eds). Proceedings of the Fourth International Tinnitus Seminar. New York, NY: Kugler Publications; 225-258.

Stypulkowski PH (1990) Mechanisms of salicylate ototoxicity. Hearing Research 46: 113-146.

Sturmey P (1996) Functional Analysis in Clinical Psychology. Chichester: John Wiley & Sons.

Sullivan M, Katon W, Russo J, Dobie R, Sakai C (1994) Coping and marital support as correlates of tinnitus disability. General Hospital Psychiatry 16: 259-266.

Sullivan MD, Katon W, Dobie R, Sakai C, Russo J, Harrop-Griffiths J (1988) Disabling tinnitus. Association with affective disorders. General Hospital Psychiatry 10: 285-291.

Sullivan MD, Katon WJ, Russo JE, Dobie RA, Sakai C (1993) A randomized trial of nortriptyline for severe chronic tinnitus. Archives of Internal Medicine 153: 2251-2259.

Surr RK, Kolb JA, Cord MT, Garrus NP (1999) Tinnitus Handicap Inventory (THI) as a hearing aid outcome measure. Journal of the American Academy of Audiology 10: 489-495.

Surr RK, Montgomery AA, Mueller HG (1985) Effect of amplification of tinnitus among new hearing aid users. Ear and Hearing 6: 71-75.

Sweetow RW (1995) The evolution of cognitive-behavioral therapy as an approach to tinnitus management. International Tinnitus Journal 1: 61-65.

Sweetow RW, Levy MC (1990) Tinnitus severity scaling for diagnostic/therapeutic usage. Hearing Instruments 41: 20-21, 46.

Szczepaniak WS, Møller AR (1996). Effects of baclofen, clonazepam and diazepam on tone exposure induced hyperexcitability of the inferior colliculus in the rat: possible therapeutic implications for pharmacological management of tinnitus and hyperacusis. Hearing Research 97: 46-53.

Terry AMP, Jones DM, Davis BR, Slater R (1983) Parametric studies of tinnitus masking and residual inhibition. British Journal of Audiology 17: 245–256.

Theopold H-M (1985) Nimodipine (Bayer 9736). A new concept in the treatment of inner ear disease. Laryngology, Rhinology and Otology 64: 609–913.

Thompson GC, Thompson AM, Garrett KM, Garrett HBB (1994) Serotonin and serotonin receptors in the central auditory system. Otolaryngology – Head and Neck Surgery 100: 93-102.

Thompson RC (1931) Assyrian prescriptions for diseases of the ear. Journal of the Royal Asiatic Society: 1–25.

Turk DC, Rudy TE, Kubinski JA, Zaki HS, Greco CM (1996) Dysfunctional patients with temporomandibular disorders: evaluating the efficacy of a tailored treatment protocol. Journal of Consulting and Clinical Psychology 64: 139–146.

Tye-Murray N (1991) Repair strategy usage by hearing-impaired adults and changes following communication therapy. Journal of Speech and Hearing Research 34: 921–928.

Tyler R, Haskell G, Preece J, Bergan C (2001) Nurturing patient expectations to enhance the treatment of tinnitus. Seminars in Hearing 22: 15–21.

Tyler RS (1984) Does tinnitus originate from hyperactive nerve fibers in the cochlea? Journal of Laryngology and Otology 9 (Suppl.): 38–44.

Tyler RS (1987) Tinnitus maskers and hearing aids for tinnitus. Seminars in Hearing 8: 49–61.

Tyler RS (1993) Tinnitus disability and handicap questionnaires. Seminars in Hearing 14: 377–383.

Tyler RS (1997) Perspectives on tinnitus. British Journal of Audiology 31: 381–386.

Tyler RS (2000) The psychoacoustical measurement of tinnitus. In: Tyler RS (ed.). Tinnitus Handbook. San Diego, Calif: Singular, Thomson Learning; 149–179.

Tyler RS, Baker LJ (1983) Difficulties experienced by tinnitus sufferers. Journal of Speech and Hearing Disorders 48: 150–154.

Tyler RS, Babin RW (1993) Tinnitus. In: Cummings CW, Frederickson JM, Harker LA, Krause CJ, Schuller DE (eds). Otolaryngology – Head and Neck Surgery. St Louis, Mich: CV Mosby; 3031–3053.

Tyler RS, Conrad-Armes D (1983a) Tinnitus pitch: a comparison of three measurement methods. British Journal of Audiology 17: 101–107.

Tyler RS, Conrad-Armes D (1983b) The determination of tinnitus loudness considering the effects of recruitment. Journal of Speech and Hearing Research 26: 59–72.

Tyler RS, Conrad-Armes D (1984) Masking of tinnitus compared to masking of pure tones. Journal of Speech and Hearing Research 27: 106–111.

Tyler RS, Stouffer JL (1989) A review of tinnitus loudness. Hearing Journal 42: 52–57.

Vallianatou N, Christodoulou P, Nestoros J, Helidonis E (2001) Audiologic and psychological profile of Greek patients with tinnitus – preliminary findings. American Journal of Otolaryngology 22: 33–37.

Vandenbroucke JP (1997) Homoeopathy trials: going nowhere. Lancet 350: 824.

Vernon J (1977) Attempts to relieve tinnitus. Journal of the American Audiology Society 2: 124–131.

Vernon J (1987a) Assessment of the tinnitus patient. In: Hazell JWPH (ed.). Tinnitus. London: Churchill Livingstone; 71–87.

Vernon JA (1987b) Pathophysiology of tinnitus: a special case – hyperacusis and a proposed treatment. American Journal of Otology 8: 201–202.

Vernon JA (Ed.) (1998) Tinnitus. Treatment and Relief. Boston, Mass: Allyn & Bacon.

Vernon JA, Meikle MB (2000) Tinnitus masking. In: Tyler RS (Ed.). Tinnitus Handbook. San Diego, Calif: Singular, Thomson Learning; 313–356.

Vernon J, Greist S, Press L (1990) Attributes of tinnitus and the acceptance of masking. American Journal of Otolaryngology 11: 44-50.

Vernon JV, Johnson R (1980) The characteristics and natural history of tinnitus in Ménière's disease. Otolaryngolic Clinics of North America 13: 611-619.

Veuillet E, Collet L, Disnat F, Morgon A (1992) Tinnitus and medial cochlear efferent system. In: Aran J-M, Dauman R, (eds). Tinitus 91. Amsterdam: Kugler; 205-209.

Viani LG (1989) Tinnitus in children with hearing loss. Journal of Laryngology and Otology 103: 142-145.

Vilholm OJ, Møller K, Jørgensen K (1998) Effect of traditional Chinese acupuncture on severe tinnitus: a double-blind, placebo-controlled, clinical investigation with open therapeutic control. British Journal of Audiology 32: 197-204.

Vlaeyen J, De Jong J, Geilen M, Heuts PHTG, Van Breukelen G (2001) Graded exposure in vivo in the treatment of pain-related fear: a replicated single-case experimental design in four patients with chronic low back pain. Behaviour Research and Therapy 39: 151-166.

Vlaeyen JW, Linton SJ (2000) Fear-avoidance and its consequences in chronic musculoskeletal pain: a state of the art. Pain 85: 317-332.

Vogt J, Kastner M (2002) Tinnituskrankungen be fluglotsen: eine klinisch–arbeitspsychologische studie. (Tinnitus in air traffic controllers: a clinical–ergonomical pilot study.) Zeitschrift fuer Arbeits und Organisationpsychologie 46: 35-44.

Wahlström B, Axelsson A (1995) The description of tinnitus sounds. In: Reich GE, Vernon JA (eds). Proceedings of the Fifth International Tinnitus Seminar. Portland, Oreg: American Tinnitus Association; 298-301.

Walger M, Von Wedel H, Hoenen S, Calero L (1998) Effectiveness of the low power laser and Ginkgo extract i.v. therapy in patients with chronic tinnitus. In: Vernon JA (ed.). Tinnitus. Treatment and Relief. Boston, Mass: Allyn & Bacon; 68-73.

Wall M, Rosenberg M, Richardson D (1987) Gaze-evoked tinnitus. Neurology 37: 1034-1036

Wallhäusser-Franke E (1997) Salicylate evokes c-fos expression in the brain stem: implications for tinnitus. NeuroReport 8: 725-728.

Wallhäusser-Franke E, Langner G (1999) Central activation patterns after experimental tinnitus induction in an animal model. In: Hazell J (ed.). Proceedings of the Sixth International Tinnitus Seminar. Cambridge: The Tinnitus and Hyperacusis Centre; 155-162.

Wallhäusser-Franke E, Braun S, Langer G (1996) Salicylate alters 2-DG uptake in the auditory system: a model for tinnitus? NeuroReport 7: 1585-1588.

Walpurger V, Hebing-Lennartz G, Denecke H, Pietrowsky R (2003) Habituation deficit in auditory event-related potentials in tinnitus complainers. Hearing Research 181: 57-64.

Walsh WM, Gerley PP (1985) Thermal biofeedback and the treatment of tinnitus. Laryngoscope 95: 987-989.

Wangemann P, Schact J (1996) Homeostatic mechanisms in the cochlea. In: Dallos P, Popper AN, Fay RR (eds). The Cochlea. New York, NY: Springer; 130-185.

Ware JE (1993) The SF36 Health Survey: Manual and Interpretation. Boston, Mass: Nimrod Press.

Wazen JJ, Foyt D, Sisti M (1997) Selective cochlear neurectomy for debilitating tinnitus. Annals of Otology, Rhinology and Laryngology 106: 568-570.

Weber C, Arck P, Mazureck B, Klapp BF (2002) Impact of relaxation training on psychometric and immunologic parameters in tinnitus sufferers. Journal of Psychosomatic Research 52: 29-33.

Weber H, Pfadenhauer K, Stohr M, Rosler A (2002) Central hyperacusis with phonophobia in multiple sclerosis. Multiple Sclerosis 8: 505–509.

Wedel von H, Calero L, Walger M, Hoenen S, Rutwalt D (1995) Soft-laser/Ginkgo Biloba therapy in chronic tinnitus. A placebo controlled study. Advances in Otorhinolaryngology 49: 105–108.

Wegel RL (1931) A study of tinnitus. Archives of Otolaryngology 14: 158–165.

Wegner DM (1994) White Bears and Other Unwanted Thoughts. New York, NY: Guilford Press.

Weinmeister KP (2000) Prolonged suppression of tinnitus after peripheral nerve block using bupivacaine and lidocaine. Regional Anesthesia and Pain Medicine 25: 67–68

Weinshel EM (1955) Some psychiatric considerations in tinnitus. Journal of the Hillside Hospital 4: 67–92.

Weinstein ND (1980) Individual differences in critical tendencies and noise annoyance. Journal of Sound and Vibration 68: 241–248.

Weir N (1990) Otolaryngology: An Illustrated History. London: Butterworths.

Weissman JL, Hirsch BE (2000) Imaging of tinnitus: a review. Radiology 216: 342–349.

Westcott M (2002) Case study: management of hyperacusis associated with post-traumatic stress disorder. In: Patuzzi R (ed.). Proceedings of the Seventh International Tinnitus Seminar. Freemantle: University of Western Australia; 280–285.

Westerberg BD, Robertson JB Jr, Stach BA (1996) A double-blind placebo-controlled trial of Baclofen in the treatment of tinnitus. American Journal of Otolaryngology 17: 896–903.

Wewers ME, Lowe NK (1990) A critical review of visual analogue scales in the measurement of clinical phenomena. Research in Nursing and Health 13: 227–236.

White TP, Hoffman SR, Gale EN (1986) Psychophysiological therapy for tinnitus. Ear and Hearing 7: 397–399.

Whittaker CK (1982) Letter to the Editor. American Journal of Otology 4: 188.

Williams JMG, Watts FN, MacLeod C, Mathews A (1997) Cognitive Psychology and Emotional Disorders. Chichester: John Wiley & Sons.

Wilson BA (1987) Rehabilitation of Memory. New York, NY: Guilford Press.

Wilson C, Lewis P, Stephens D (2002) The short form 36 (SF 36) in a specialist tinnitus clinic. International Journal of Audiology 41: 216–220.

Wilson J, Sutton GJ (1981) Acoustic correlates of tonal tinnitus. In: Evered D, Lawrenson G (eds). Tinnitus, Ciba Foundation Symposium 85. London: Pitman Books; 82–100.

Wilson PH, Henry JL (1998) Tinnitus cognitions questionnaire: development and psychometric properties of a measure of dysfunctional cognitions associated with tinnitus. International Tinnitus Journal 4: 23–30.

Wilson PH, Henry J, Bowen M, Haralambous G (1991) Tinnitus reaction questionnaire: psychometric properties of a measure of distress associated with tinnitus. Journal of Speech and Hearing Research 34: 197–201.

Wilson PH, Henry JL, Andersson G, Hallam RS, Lindberg P (1998) A critical analysis of directive counselling as a component of tinnitus retraining therapy. British Journal of Audiology 32: 273–286.

Wise K, Rief W, Goebel G (1998) Meeting the expectations of chronic tinnitus patients: comparison of a structured group therapy program for tinnitus management with a problem-solving group. Journal of Psychosomatic Research 44: 681–685.

WHO (1980) International Classification of Impairments, Disabilities and Handicaps. Geneva: World Health Organization.

WHO (2001). International Classification of Functioning, Disability and Health. Geneva: World Health Organization.

Wood KA, Webb WL, Orchik DJ, Shea JJ (1983) Intractable tinnitus: psychiatric aspects of treatment. Psychosomatics 24: 559-565.

Woodhouse A, Drummond PD (1993) Mechanisms of increased sensitivity to noise and light in migraine headache. Cephalgia 13: 417-421.

Wright EF, Bifano SL (1997) Tinnitus improvement through TMD therapy. Journal of the American Dental Association 128: 1424-1432.

Yetiser S, Tosun F, Satar B, Arslanhan M, Akcam T, Ozakaptan Y (2002) The role of zinc in management of tinnitus. Auris Nasus Larynx 29: 329-333.

Young DW (2000) Biofeedback training in the treatment of tinnitus. In: Tyler RS (ed.). Tinnitus Handbook. San Diego, Calif: Singular, Thomson Learning; 281-295.

Zachariae R, Mirz F, Johansen LV, Andersen SE, Bjerring P, Pedersen CB (2000) Reliability and validity of a Danish adaption of the tinnitus handicap inventory. Scandinavian Audiology 29: 37-43.

Zatorre RJ, Binder JR (2000) Functional and structural imaging of the human auditory system. In: Toga AW, Mazziotta JC (eds). Brain Mapping. The Systems. San Diego, Calif: Academic Press; 365-402.

Zelman S (1973) Correlation of smoking history with hearing loss. Journal of the American Medical Association 233: 920.

Zenner HP, Ernst A (1993) Cochlear-motor, transduction and signal-transfer tinnitus: models for three types of cochlear tinnitus. European Archives of Otorhinolaryngology 249: 447-454.

Zhang JS, Kaltenbach JA (1998) Increases in spontaneous activity in the dorsal cochlear nucleus of the rat following exposure to high intensity sound. Neuroscience Letters 250: 197-200.

Zigmond AS, Snaith RP (1983) The hospital anxiety and depression scale. Acta Psychiatrica Scandinavia 67: 361-370.

Zimmer K, Ellermeier W (1999) Psychometric properties of four measures of noise sensitivity: a comparison. Journal of Environmental Psychology 19: 295-302.

Zöger S, Holgers K-M, Svedlund J (2001) Psychiatric disorders in tinnitus patients without severe hearing impairment: 24 month follow-up of patients at an audiological clinic. Audiology 40: 133-140.

Index

acoustic neurinoma *see* vestibular schwannoma
acoustic neuroma *see* vestibular schwannoma
acupuncture 160-161
alcohol 36, 98, 109-110
alprazolam 126
altered neural activity 29-30
alternative medicine 159 (*see also* complementary medicine)
aminoglycoside 35-36
amino-oxyacetic acid 127
amitriptyline 126
animal models 29-30
antiepileptic drugs 127
anti-malarial drugs 35
antispasmodic drugs 127
anxiety 90, 94-95, 98-100, 104, 107
anxiety sensitivity 102
arachidonic acid 29, 36
aromatherapy 162
associative learning 58
attention 61
attention-diversion techniques 149
auditory system
    cerebellopontine angle 9-10
    cochlea 7
    inner hair cells 8
    internal auditory canal 9
    middle ear 6-7
    outer ear   5
    outer hair cells 8
    spiral ganglion 9
    tympanic membrane 5-6
    see also central auditory pathways

auditory brainstem audiometry 72
autobiographical memories 100
autonomic nervous system 57-58, 135
autonomic nervous system arousal 95

baclofen 127
Beck Depression Inventory 94
benign intracranial hypertension 45-46
benzodiazepines 126
betahistine 127
biofeedback 130-131
Brodmann map 76
bupivicaine 125

caffeine 109-110
calcium 27-29
calcium transport 27
calmodulin 28
candles, hopi ear 164
cannabis 36
carbamazepine 127
carotid stenosis 45
caroverine 127
catastrophic thinking 107, 152
CBT *see* cognitive behavioural therapy
central auditory pathways
    associative cortices 12
    cochlear nucleus 10-11
    inferior colliculus 11-12, 79
    medial geniculate body 12
    medial olivo-cochlear bundle 11
    superior olivary complex 11
changing state 60-62, 100
chemodectoma *see* glomus tumour

children
    normal hearing children and tinnitus
        20
    role of hearing impairment 20
    sleep problems 97
    tinnitus experiences 93
    tinnitus prevalence 19–20
chronic suppurative otitis media 39
CIDI-SF 95
ciprofloxacin 35
cisplatin 35
classical conditioning 58, 119, 138
classification schemes 82–84
clinical significance of treatment 155
cobalamin 162
cochlea 7
cochlear implantation 129–130
cognitive behavioural therapy (CBT),
    case-formulation 148
    cognitive methods 152
    compared with TRT 140
    concentration 149
    definition of 145
    distraction methods 149
    evaluation 157
    evidence 154
    exposure 149
    internet 153–4, 157
    need for supervision 157
    relapse prevention 152
    sleep management 150
    use in hyperacusis 121
Cognitive Failures Questionnaire 91, 99
cognitive function 61, 99–100
cognitive therapy 152
combination instruments 129
complementary medicine 159–165
Composite International Diagnostic
    Interview – Short Form (CIDI-SF) 95
concentration problems 93
conductive hearing loss 36–39, 45
chronic suppurative otitis media 39
    otosclerosis 36–38
    secretory otitis media 39
contiguity 58
Controlled Word Association Test 100
coping 101, 106–107
coping strategies 145
coping style 106–107
core professional knowledge 168
cortical reorganization 32

Costen's syndrome 50
craniofacial disorder see temporo-
        mandibular disorder
CSOM see chronic suppurative otitis
        media
cyclo-oxygenase 29, 36
cytotoxic drugs 35

Deafness see hearing impairment
definitions,
    tinnitus 1, 2,
    hyperacusis 2, 112
depression 90, 94, 100, 104–105, 107
Diagnostic and Statistical Manual of Mental
        Disorders (DSM) 94
diaries 84, 156
diathesis-stress 101, 146
diazepam 126
dietary supplements 162–163
    vitamins 162
    minerals 163
    zinc 163
    magnesium 163
directive counselling 136 138
discordant damage hypothesis 25–26
distraction 149
diuretics 128
dizziness 102
drug-induced tinnitus 35–36
    anti-inflammatory drugs 35
    antibiotics 35–36
    antimalarian agents 35
    salicylates 35–36
    recreational drugs 36
DSM-III-R see Diagnostic and
        Statistical Manual of Mental
        Disorders
DSM-IV see Diagnostic and Statistical
        Manual of Mental Disorders
dual task 99
dynorphins 29, 119

earplugs 120
ecstasy 36
effect size 154
electrical stimulation 129–130
    transdermic electrical nerve stimulation
        129
    cochlear implantation 78, 129–130
emotional distress 93–96
endolymphatic hydrops 40–41

environmental conditions 110
ephatic coupling 32, 43–44
eustachian tube, patulous 49
evaluative conditioning 60
evoked potentials 72
evoked response audiometry 72
Eysenck Personality Questionnaire
        105–106

facial nerve dysfunction 116
family 90, 108
    spouse reactions 108
    attachment patterns 109
Family Support Scale 91
frusemide *see* furosemide
furosemide 35, 128
functional magnetic resonance imaging
        (fMRI) 73

GABA *see also* gamma aminobutyric acid
gamma aminobutyric acid 126
gaze-evoked tinnitus 32, 77, 79
gender differences 102
General Health Questionnaire 94
gentamicin, intratympanic 41
ginkgo biloba 161
glomus tumour 45, 49
glue ear *see* secretory otitis media
glutamate 29, 119
glycerol 128

habituation 107, 146
habituation model 55–56, 58–60
hearing impairment 82, 84, 90, 95,
        99–100, 103, 107
hearing aids 103, 128, 138
hearing tactics 151
help-*seek*ing 23
history,
    of tinnitus 2–4
    of treatments 2–4
homeopathy 160
hopi ear candles 164
Hospital Anxiety and Depression Scale 90,
        95, 157
hyperacusis, 112–122
    auditory efferent dysfunction 118 – 119
    Bells palsy 117
    borrelia burgdorferi 117
    causes 116–120
    classical conditioning model 119

cochlear blood flow 118
cognitive behavioural therapy 121–122
coincident with tinnitus 114
definition 2, 112
depression 113 117
desensitization 121
dynorphins 119
earplugs 120
fear avoidance model 119–120
fear conditionong 118
glutamate 119
head injury 117
5 hydroxytryptamine 118
5-HT 117 118
Lyme disease 117 121
measurement of
mechanisms 116–118
migraine 113, 117–118
multiple sclerosis 117
outer hair cells 118
perilymph fistula 117
post-traumatic stress disorder 117, 118
prevalence 114–115
psychiatric disease 114
psychological model 119
Ramsey Hunt syndrome 117
reticular formation 118–119
self-report 116
serotonin 113, 118
sound generators 121
stapedectomy 117
stapedial reflex 116
ticks 117
tinnitus retraining therapy 121–122
treatment 120–122
vestibular nerve section 119
William's syndrome 117 118
hypericum perforatum 162
hypnotherapy 132–133
hypozincaemia 163
hysteria 106

ICF *see* International Classification of
        Functioning Disability and Health
IHC *see* inner hair cells
imagery 149
inner hair cells 8
insomnia *see* sleep disturbance
Insomnia Severity Index 90–91
International Classification of Functioning
        Disability and Health   92

internet,
    epidemiology 115
    self-help 153-154
    treatment 156
    use in diagnosis 94
intratympanic gentamicin 41

laser 163-164
leukotriene 36
lidocaine 76-78, 125
Life Orientation Scale 105
life-time diagnosis 94
lignocaine see also lidocaine
limbic system 13, 59, 135
local anaesthetic drugs 124-5
localization 22
locus of control 107-108
longitudinal studies of tinnitus 21-22
loop diuretic 35
lorazepam 126
loudness measures 66
    hearing level 66
    sensation level 66
    recruitment 67, 112, 114
loudness recruitment 112-114
Lyme disease 117

magnesium 163
magnetic stimulation 163
magnetic resonance imaging 42, 73
mannitol 128
maskability 67
    Feldmann's masking curves 69
minimal masking level 67, 102
    narrow-band noise 68
    test-retest reliability 70
    tinnitus masking curves 68
    white noise 68
masking as treatment 60, 128-129, 150
    combination instruments 129
    hearing aids 128
masking devices 128
    placebo 128
medial olivo-cochlear system 11
medial efferent system 30-31
meditation 162
melatonin 162
memory 60
Ménière's disease 39-42
    endolymphatic hydrops 40-41
    incidence 40
    intratympanic gentamicin 41

labyrinthectomy 42
    management 40-42
    prevalence 40
    surgery 41
    vestibular nerve section 42
meta-analysis 131, 154, 166
mineral supplements 162 163
Minnesota Multiphasic Personality
        Inventory 105-106
misophonia 113
mixing point 138-139
moderating factors 101-102
mood disorder 95
MRI see magnetic resonance imaging
multidisciplinary teams 167-168
multiple sclerosis 117
myoclonus 47
    middle ear myoclonus 47
    palatal myoclonus 47
    tensor tympani syndrome 47

N-methyl-D-asparatate receptors 29
neurophysiological model 56-59, 101,
        103, 135-136
niacin 162
nimodipine 127
NMDA receptors 29
noise annoyance 113-114
noise sensitivity 113-114, 116
non-steroidal anti-inflammatory drugs 35
normal hearing   26
nortriptyline 126
NSAIDs   35

OHC see outer hair cells
Old age and tinnitus 20-21
OME see secretory otitis media
open-ended approaches 89
opioid receptors 29
optimism 105
oral facial movement 77
osmotic diuretics 128
otitis media with effusion see secretory
        otitis media
otoacoustic emissions 26-27, 31, 50
otoacoustic emissions, spontaneous 50
otosclerosis 36-38
    aetiology 37
    fenestration 38
    fluoride 38
    genetics 37
    incidence 37

mobilization 38
prevalence 37
pulsatile tinnitus 37
stapedectomy 38
treatment 38
ototoxicity 25, 30 *see also* also drug
  induced tinnitus
outer hair cells 8, 118

pain analogy 31-32
palatal myoclonus 47
patient categories in Tinnitus Retraining
  Therapy 137
patulous eustachian tube 49
Pavlov's experiments 58
perfectionism 102
personality 105-106
PET *see* positron emission
  tomography
phantom limb pain 32
Pharmacological treatment of tinnitus
  alprazolam 126
  amino-oxyacetic acid 127
  amitriptyline 126
  anaesthetic drugs 124-125
  antiepileptic drugs 127
  antispasmodic drugs 127
  baclofen 127
  benzodiazepines 126
  betahistine 127
  bupivicaine 125
  calcium channels 127
  carbamazepine 127
  caroverine 127
  diazepam 126
  diuretics 128
  frusemide *see also* furosemide
  furosemide 128
  GABA *see* gamma aminobutyric
    acid
  gamma aminobutyric acid 126
  glycerol 128
  intra-tympanic 125
  lamotrigine 127
  lidocaine 125
  lignocaine *see also* lidocaine
  local anaesthetic drugs 124-5
  lorazepam 126
  mannitol 128
  nimodipine 127
  nortriptyline 126
  osmotic diuretics 128

procaine 125
  selective serotonin reuptake inhibitor
    126
  serotonin 125
  sodium channels 125-127
  SSRI *see* selective serotonin reuptake
    inhibitor
  tocainide 125
  tricyclic antidepressants 126
  trimipramine 126
  vasodilators 127
phonophobia 113-114
pitch matching 65
positron emission tomography (PET) 73,
  76
placebo 159-160, 164-165
precuneus 77, 80
prevalence,
  prolonged spontaneous tinnitus 14
  transient tinnitus 14
  Heller and Bergman experiment 15
  prevalence studies 15-19
  life-time tinnitus 19
  incidence 19
  natural history 21
procaine 125
profound sensorineural hearing loss 26
prostaglandins 29, 36
psychoacoustic measures 95
psychoanalysis 133
psychodynamic therapy 133
psychological assessment 147-148
pulsatile tinnitus 45-48
  atherosclerosis 45
  benign intracranial hypertension 45-46
  carotid stenosis 45
  conductive hearing loss 45
  glomus tumour 45, 49
  investigation 46-47, 48
  investigation algorithm 48
  management 47
pyridoxine 162

Quality of Family Life Questionnaire 91
questionnaires 86-91
quinine 28-29, 35

randomised controlled trials 166
reaction time 71
recreational drugs 36
recruitment *see also* loudness recruitment
reflexology 162

relapse 152
relaxation therapy 131–132, 150, 159
    applied relaxation 131, 148
    passive relaxation 131
    progressive relaxation 149
    rapid relaxation 149
    yoga 132
repetitive transcranial magnetic
        stimulation 80
residual inhibition 69
reticular formation 13, 57
ribosomes 36

Saint John's wort 162
salicylates 28–30 35–36
self help 153–154, 157
self-hypnosis 132
self-report measures 84,
    Cognitive Failures Questionnaire 91, 99
    Hospital Anxiety and Depression Scale
        90, 95, 157
    Insomnia Severity Index 90–91
    Short Form 36 (SF-36) 90–91
    Subjective Tinnitus Severity Scale 87, 88
    Tinnitus Coping Strategy Questionnaire
        89
    Tinnitus Coping Style Questionnaire 89
    Tinnitus Handicap Inventory 87, 89, 91,
        106
    Tinnitus Handicap Questionnaire 88
    Tinnitus Questionnaire 87, 88, 90, 91
    Tinnitus Reaction Questionnaire 86, 88,
        106
    Tinnitus Severity Scale 87, 88
serotonin (5-HT) 32–33, 117, 125
SF 36 see also Short Form 36
Short Form 36, 90–91
single photon emission computed tomog-
        raphy (SPECT) 73
sleep disturbance 90, 93, 97–99, 147, 150,
        155, 156
    prevalence 98
    cognitive behavioural model 98
sleep management 150
smoking 109–110
SOAE see spontaneous otoacoustic
        emissions
sodium channels 125, 127
somatic modulation 31, 148
somatic problems 102

somatosensory 31
sound enrichment 139, 150
sound generators 136 137–9
sound therapy 136
sound quality 63–65
    examples of sounds 65
    metaphor 64
spiral ganglion 9
spontaneous activity 30
spontaneous otoacoustic emissions 50
SSNHL see sudden sensorineural hearing
        loss
SSRI see selective serotonin reuptake
        inhibitor
stapedectomy 38
stapedius, myoclonus of 47
startle response 113
stimulation
    electrical 129–130
    laser 163–164
    magnetic 163
    ultrasonic 163
stocastic resonance 33, 43
stress 103–104, 119
Stroop test 99
structured interviews 84, 147
Subjective Tinnitus Severity Scale 87, 88
sudden sensorineural hearing loss 51–53
    investigations 53
    treatment protocol 52–53
suicide 96–97
sufi proverb 166
surgical treatment of tinnitus
    cochlear implantation 129–130
    cochlear neurectomy 123–4
    decompression of auditory nerve 124
    destructive procedures 123
    Ménière's disease 41–42
    non-syndromic tinnitus 123–4
    otosclerosis 38
    vestibular schwannoma 44
synthesizers 65–66

temporomandibular disorder 50–51
    Costen's syndrome 50
    diagnosis 50
    management 51
stomatognatic treatment 51
    temporomandibular joint arthroscopy
        51

tensor tympani syndrome 47
tensor tympani, myoclonus of 47
THI *see* Tinnitus Handicap Inventory
thiamine 162
thought stopping 149
Tinnitus Cognitions Questionnaire 89
Tinnitus Coping Strategy Questionnaire 89
Tinnitus Coping Style Questionnaire 89
Tinnitus Handicap Inventory 87, 89, 91,
      106
Tinnitus Handicap Questionnaire 87, 88,
      106
Tinnitus Handicap/Support Scale 87, 88
Tinnitus Questionnaire 87, 89, 90, 91
Tinnitus Reaction Questionnaire 86, 88
      106
tinnitus retraining therapy (TRT) 59,
      135-144
   autonomic nervous system 135
   clinical protocol 136-139
   cognitive therapy 136
   combination instruments 138
   critique 136, 140-141
   directive counselling 136 138
   evidence for efficacy 139-140 142-143
   hearing aids 138
   limbic system 135
   mixing point 138-9
   neurophysiological model 56-59, 101,
      103, 135-136
   patient categories 137-138
   protocol 136
   sound enrichment 139, 150
   sound generators 136 137-139
   sound therapy 136
   use in hyperacusis 121
Tinnitus Severity Scale 87, 88

TMJ dysfunction *see* temporomandibular
      disorder
tocainide 125
tonotopic reorganization 30
TRT *see* tinnitus retraining therapy
tricyclic antidepressants 126
trimipramine 126

ultrasonic stimulation 163

vasodilators 127
vestibular nerve section 42, 119
vestibular schwannomas 42-44
   cochlear tinnitus 44
   ephaptic coupling 43, 44
   incidence 42-43
   management 44
   pre- and postoperative tinnitus 43
   radiotherapy 44
   stereotactic radiotherapy (gamma knife)
      44
   surgery 44
   stochastic resonance 43
visual analogue scale 84
vitamin B 162-163
vitamin supplements 162-163

WHO *see* World Health Organization
Williams syndrome 117
World Health Organization 92
work 100, 152
working memory 60

yoga 132, 162

zinc 163